Study Guide

Leifer

Introduction to Maternity & Pediatric Nursing

Fifth Edition

Emily Slone McKinney, MSN, RNC
Baylor Healthcare System
Women and Children's Services
Dallas, Texas

Christine M. Rosner, RN, PhD
Dean
School of Nursing and Allied Health Professions
Holy Family University
Philadelphia, Pennsylvania

SAUNDERS

ELSEVIER

SAUNDERS
ELSEVIER

11830 Westline Industrial Drive
St. Louis, Missouri 63146

Introduction to Maternity and Pediatric Nursing, 5th edition

ISBN-13: 978-1-4160-4682-0
ISBN-10: 1-4160-4682-8

Notice

Nursing is an ever-changing field. Standard safety precautions must be followed, but as new research and clinical experience broaden our knowledge, changes in treatment and drug therapy may become necessary or appropriate. Readers are advised to check the most current product information provided by the manufacturer of each drug to be administered to verify the recommended dose, the method, and duration of administration, and contraindications. It is the responsibility of the licensed prescriber, relying on experience and knowledge of the patient, to determine dosages and the best treatment for each individual patient. Neither the publisher nor the author assume any liability for any injury and/or damage to persons or property arising from this publication.

The Publisher

ISBN-13: 978-1-4160-4682-0
ISBN-10: 1-4160-4682-8

Acquisitions Editor: Robin Levin Richman
Developmental Editor: Ryan Creed
Publishing Services Manager: Gayle May
Project Manager: Tracey Schriefer

Printed in the United States of America
Last digit is the print number: 9 8 7 6 5 4 3 2

Preface

This Study Guide is written to promote student mastery of *Introduction to Maternity & Pediatric Nursing*, Fifth Edition, by Gloria Leifer. Each chapter in this Study Guide corresponds to the text chapter having the same number and title.

The authors have included matching and completion **Learning Activities** to help students learn basic factual knowledge that underlies nursing care. Other exercises request the student to list or describe text information to encourage reading comprehension and written expression of what is learned. Labeling of illustrations is included to help the student understand anatomy, as appropriate.

To promote higher level learning, the authors have included **Thinking Critically** activities, which ask the student to apply knowledge or draw conclusions based on material in the textbook but not directly answered in the textbook. **Case Studies** and **Applying Knowledge** activities provide ideas for applying factual content to client care.

Each chapter contains multiple choice **Review Questions**. The questions ask for appropriate nursing actions, what the nurse should expect in terms of medical orders or usual care of the client, and what complication the client is at risk of developing, as well as items that review basic factual information from the chapter. Some chapters conclude with **Crossword Puzzles** to further test comprehension of terms and concepts.

An answer key for the Learning Activities, selected Thinking Critically activities, Review Questions, and Crossword Puzzles has been provided for your instructor.

To the Student

This Study Guide was created to assist you in achieving the objectives of each chapter in *Introduction to Maternity & Pediatric Nursing*, Fifth Edition, and establishing a solid base of knowledge in maternity and pediatric nursing. Completing the exercises in each chapter in this Guide will help to reinforce the material studied in the textbook and learned in class. Such reinforcement also helps students to be successful on the NCLEX-PN®.

Study Hints for All Students

Ask Questions!

There are no stupid questions. If you do not know something or are not sure, you need to find out. Other people may be wondering the same thing but may be too shy to ask. The answer could mean life or death to your patient. That is certainly more important than feeling embarrassed about asking a question.

Chapter Objectives

At the beginning of each chapter in the textbook are objectives that you should have mastered when you finish studying that chapter. Write these objectives in your notebook, leaving a blank space after each. Fill in the answers as you find them while reading the chapter. Review to make sure your answers are correct and complete. Use these answers when you study for tests. This should also be done for separate course objectives that your instructor has listed in your class syllabus.

Key Terms

At the beginning of each chapter in the textbook are key terms that you will encounter as you read the chapter. Text page number references are provided, for easy reference and review, and the key terms are in color the first time they appear in the chapter. Phonetic pronunciations are provided for terms that students might find difficult to pronounce. The terms that were assigned simple phonetic pronunciations were selected because they are either (1) difficult medical, nursing, or scientific terms or (2) other words that may be difficult for students to pronounce. The goal is to help the student reader with limited proficiency in English to develop a greater command of the pronunciation of scientific and nonscientific English terminology. It is hoped that a more general competency in the understanding and use of medical and scientific language may result.

Key Points

Use the Key Points at the end of each chapter in the textbook to help with review for exams.

Reading Hints

When reading each chapter in the textbook, look at the subject headings to learn what each section is about. Read first for the general meaning. Then reread parts you did not understand. It may help to read those parts aloud. Carefully read the information given in each table and study each figure and its caption.

Concepts

While studying, put difficult concepts into your own words to see if you understand them. Check this understanding with another student or the instructor. Write these in your notebook.

Class Notes

When taking lecture notes in class, leave a large margin on the left side of each notebook page and write only on right-hand pages, leaving all left-hand pages blank. Look over your lecture notes soon after each class, while your memory is fresh. Fill in missing words, complete sentences and ideas, and underline key phrases, definitions, and concepts. At the top of each page, write the topic of that page. In the left margin, write the key word for that part of your notes. On the opposite left-hand page, write a summary or outline that combines material from both the textbook and the lecture. These can be your study notes for review.

Study Groups

Form a study group with some other students so you can help one another. Practice speaking and reading aloud. Ask questions about material you are not sure about. Work together to find answers.

References for Improving Study Skills

Good study skills are essential for achieving your goals in nursing. Time management, efficient use of study time, and a consistent approach to studying are all beneficial. There are various study methods for reading a textbook and for taking class notes. Some methods that have proven helpful can be found in *Saunders Student Nurse Planner: A Guide to Success in Nursing School.* This book contains helpful information on test-taking and preparing for clinical experiences. It includes an example of a "time map" for planning study time and a blank form that the student can use to formulate a personal time map.

Additional Study Hints for English as a Second Language (ESL) Students

Vocabulary

If you find a nontechnical word you do not know (e.g., *drowsy*), try to guess its meaning from the sentence; e.g., *With electrolyte imbalance, the patient may feel fatigued and drowsy.* If you are not sure of the meaning, or if it seems particularly important, look it up in the dictionary.

Vocabulary Notebook

Keep a small alphabetized notebook or address book in your pocket or purse. Write down new nontechnical words you read or hear along with their meanings and pronunciations. Write each word under its initial letter so you can find it easily, as in a dictionary. For words you do not know or for words that have a different meaning in nursing, write down how they are used and sound. Look up their meanings in a dictionary or ask your instructor or first-language buddy. Then write the different meanings or usages that you have found in your book, including the nursing meaning. Continue to add new words as you discover them. For example:

primary	•	of most importance; main: *the primary problem or disease*
	•	the first one; elementary: *primary school*
secondary	•	of less importance; resulting from another problem or disease: *a secondary symptom*
	•	the second one: *secondary school (in the United States, high school)*

First-Language Buddy

ESL students should find a first-language buddy—another student who is a native speaker of English and who is willing to answer questions about word meanings, pronunciations, and culture. Maybe your buddy would like to learn about your language and culture as well. This could help in his or her nursing experience also.

Contents

CHAPTER 1

Student Name _____

The Past, Present, and Future

Answer Key: Textbook page references are provided as a guide for answering these questions. A complete answer key was provided for your instructor.

LEARNING ACTIVITIES

1. Match the terms in the left column with their definitions on the right (a–i).

   _____ Advanced practice nurse *(12)*

   _____ Clinical pathways *(6)*

   _____ Diagnosis-related groups (DRG) *(11)*

   _____ Empowerment *(2)*

   _____ Family-centered care *(2)*

   _____ Health maintenance organization (HMO) *(11)*

   _____ Managed care *(11)*

   _____ Preferred provider organization (PPO) *(11)*

   _____ Variance *(6)*

   a. The difference between the expected outcome and the outcome achieved

   b. Recognizing the strength and integrity of the family as the core of planning and implementing health care

   c. A registered nurse with an advanced degree who specializes in a clinical area of nursing such as obstetrics or pediatrics and may conduct research in their specialty

   d. A system used by government-financed programs that determines payment for a person's hospital stay based on the diagnosis

   e. A health organization that contracts with providers for services at a discount for its members

   f. A health care delivery system that contracts with providers to provide services at a fixed capitated fee each month

   g. An organization that offers health services for a fixed premium

   h. Research-based guidelines for expected progress within a timeline

   i. Providing the means by which families accept and maintain control over their members' health care

2. List three health care professionals who deliver babies. *(1-2)*

   a. _____

   b. _____

   c. _____

3. Match the names in the left column with their contributions toward improvement of maternal, newborn, and pediatric care on the right (a–j).

_____ Samuel Bard *(2)*

_____ Karl Credé *(2)*

_____ Abraham Jacobi *(3)*

_____ Oliver Wendell Holmes *(2)*

_____ Joseph Lister *(2)*

_____ Louis Pasteur *(2)*

_____ Margaret Sanger *(17)*

_____ Ignaz Semmelweis *(2)*

_____ Soranus *(2)*

_____ Lillian Wald *(3-4, 17)*

a. Associated unwashed hands of medical students following dissection of cadavers and puerperal fever among postpartum women

b. Determined that puerperal fever was caused by bacteria that could be spread by people and objects

c. Helped establish the Children's Bureau, leading to birth registration and school lunch programs

d. Developed a treatment to prevent infant blindness caused by gonorrhea

e. Wrote a paper about the contagiousness of puerperal fever, thus initiating the germ theory of disease

f. Wrote the first American textbook on obstetrics for midwives

g. Applied antiseptic principles to surgical practice

h. Introduced podalic version to deliver the second twin

i. Established pediatric nursing as a medical specialty

j. Provided care for poor pregnant women that was the seed for development of today's Planned Parenthood programs

4. List three professional organizations concerned with maternity nursing. *(3)*

a. _____

b. _____

c. _____

5. Describe how each listed governmental program influences maternity and pediatric care.

a. Title V Amendment of the Social Security Act *(3)*

_____

_____

b. Title XIX of the Medicaid program *(3)*

_____

_____

Student Name_____

    c. Head Start program *(3)*

_____

_____

    d. National Center for Family Planning *(3)*

_____

_____

    e. Women's, Infant's, and Children's program *(3)*

_____

_____

    f. Family and Medical Leave Act (FMLA) *(3)*

_____

_____

    g. Fair Labor Standards Act *(5)*

_____

_____

    h. Education for All Handicapped Children Act *(5)*

_____

_____

    i. Missing Children's Act *(5)*

_____

_____

6. How has the inpatient stay for birth changed recently? What implication do you believe these changes have for nurses? *(6)*

_____

_____

7. How have consumers changed practices in maternity care? *(7)*

_____

_____

8. Give examples of how technology and development of medical specialties affects the care of infants and children. *(9-10)*

_____

_____

_____

_____

9. How have advances in technology contributed to the growing population of chronically ill children? *(11)*

_____

_____

10. Give two examples of advanced practice nurses. *(11-12)*

a. _____

b. _____

11. List the steps of the nursing process. *(12)*

a. _____

b. _____

c. _____

d. _____

e. _____

f. _____

12. What is the place of the Nursing Interventions Classification (NIC) and Nursing Outcome Criteria (NOC) in patient care and reimbursement for nursing services? *(14-15)*

_____

_____

_____

_____

13. Explain the meaning and use of critical thinking in nursing. *(14)*

_____

_____

Student Name_____

14. What is *Healthy People 2010?* *(16)*

_____

_____

APPLYING KNOWLEDGE

1. What is the typical hospital stay for a woman who has an uncomplicated vaginal birth at your clinical facility? For a woman who has an uncomplicated cesarean birth? Do insurance companies or HMOs offer home visits to women who had uncomplicated births? Ask nurses how they manage their care to accommodate short postpartum hospital stays.

2. Talk with a father who was present at the birth of his child. How did the experience affect him? If he has more than one child and was not present at all the births, does he perceive any differences in how he feels toward his children based on whether he was present at their births?

3. When you are in the clinical area, care for a childbearing family from a cultural group other than your own. Use the assessment questions listed under "Cross-Cultural Considerations" in your text to better understand the family's views toward birth.

4. When you are in the clinical area, observe how the family is involved in the birth process. Talk to new grandparents about how birth has changed since their children were born. Use the following questions as a springboard to discussion or answer them alone.
   a. Were you involved in the birth of your children? What pain relief was available where you gave birth?
   b. How do you feel about the involvement of fathers in childbirth?
   c. How do cultural influences seem to affect women and their families when birth occurs? Do you see differences between new immigrant families and those who have been in our country for more than one generation?
   d. Do you think siblings of the new baby should be involved during or after birth? If so, in what way?

5. Ask the birth facility in your clinical area what types of statistical data they gather and what is done with that data. Use www.cdc.gov/nchs to locate the most recent information about number of births, term births, preterm births, and low birth weight infants. What are the percentages of cesarean births and vaginal births during the most recent year at your clinical facility?

6. Does your clinical facility use a method of computerized charting? What security measures assure privacy of a patient's data? What arrangements does the facility have if the computer system is down?

7. List ways that you use critical thinking to solve problems or meet needs in daily non-nursing aspects of your life.

REVIEW QUESTIONS

1. The Credé method prevents newborn eye infection by use of: *(2)*
   1. antibiotic ointment.
   2. silver nitrate solution.
   3. washing each eye separately.
   4. using gloves for all care.

2. The most important nursing action to prevent infection in any patient is to: *(2)*
   1. use disposable equipment.
   2. consistently wash your hands.
   3. limit visitors to family members.
   4. wear hospital-laundered clothes.

3. To best improve the care of a pregnant woman from a different cultural group, the nurse should: *(7)*
   1. identify the woman's expectations about pregnancy and birth.
   2. observe the woman and her family as they interact.
   3. learn about members of different local cultural groups.
   4. encourage the woman to adopt local childbearing practices.

4. One way in which nurses may use statistics is to: *(7-9)*
   1. determine daily staffing to maintain the best patient care.
   2. predict the hospital census for the following year.
   3. evaluate the outcomes of prenatal care provided.
   4. compute the number of women who conceive each year.

5. Choose the care that best describes use of critical thinking in nursing care. *(15-16)*
   1. Maintaining the principles of sterile technique when performing catheterization of a woman with her leg in a cast
   2. Assessing the likelihood of a woman being abused while her family is present
   3. Identifying how statistical information can be used to plan a research project
   4. Looking up all medications and their doses before administering them to adults and/or children

6. Choose the best description of certified nurse-midwife (CNM) qualifications. *(7)*
   1. Gives limited care to women after normal childbirth.
   2. Assists in the prenatal care of high-risk women.
   3. Primarily provides care to low-income women.
   4. Attends uncomplicated births of low-risk women.

7. The nursing process is best described as a method to: *(12-14)*
   1. identify patients who have an increased risk for medical complications.
   2. reduce the incidence of complications for expectant mothers and infants.
   3. identify and solve patient problems with individualized nursing care.
   4. promote breastfeeding in groups that do not usually nurse infants.

8. Choose the best description for a variance in a clinical pathway. *(6)*
   1. The patient did not cooperate with the recommended therapy.
   2. An achieved patient outcome differs from the expected outcome.
   3. Patient care is individualized, appropriate to a specific person.
   4. Reimbursement will be curtailed because of a complication.

CHAPTER 2

Student Name _____

Human Reproductive Anatomy and Physiology

Answer Key: Textbook page references are provided as a guide for answering these questions. A complete answer key was provided for your instructor.

LEARNING ACTIVITIES

1. _____ is the time when reproductive systems mature and become capable of reproduction. *(19)*

2. Hormonal changes of puberty in boys begin between the ages of _____ and _____ years. The first outward male changes of puberty are growth of the _____ and _____. *(19)*

3. The first outward change of puberty in girls is _____ . The first menstrual period usually occurs _____ after this initial change. *(19-20)*

4. Describe secondary sexual characteristics in boys and girls. *(19-20)*

    a. Boys _____

    _____

    b. Girls _____

    _____

5. Match the terms in the left column with their definitions on the right (a–h).

_____	Androgens *(20)*	a. Organs that produce spermatozoa and male sex hormones
_____	Penis *(20)*	b. Seminal plasma plus sperm
_____	Scrotum *(20)*	c. Male sex hormones
_____	Semen *(21)*	d. Primary male hormone
_____	Spermatogenesis *(20)*	e. Male germ (reproductive) cells
_____	Spermatozoa *(20)*	f. Male organ for urination and sexual intercourse
_____	Testes *(20)*	g. Production of spermatozoa
_____	Testosterone *(20)*	h. Skin sac that suspends testes away from the body

6.   Label the structures of the male reproductive system on the figure below. *(20-21)*

a.   Anus
b.   Bulbourethral gland
c.   Ejaculatory duct
d.   Epididymis
e.   Foreskin of penis
f.   Glans penis
g.   Penis

h.   Prostate gland
i.   Scrotum
j.   Seminal vesicle
k.   Testis
l.   Urethra
m.   Urinary bladder
n.   Vas deferens

7.   a.   Spermatozoa are produced in the _____ of the testes. *(20)*
     b.   Testosterone is produced in the _____ of the testes. *(20)*

8.   Describe six effects of testosterone. *(20-21)*

a.   _____

b.   _____

c.   _____

d.   _____

e.   _____

f.   _____

Student Name _____

9.   Label the structures of the external female genitalia on the figure below. *(21)*

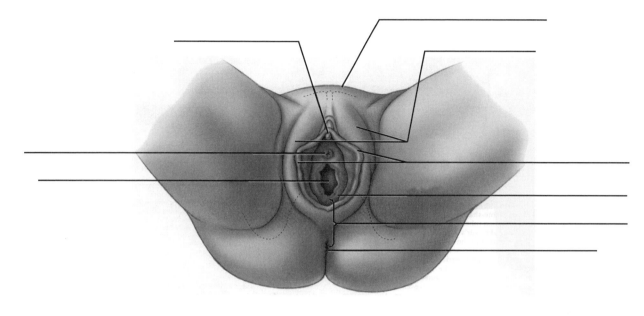

a.   Anus
b.   Clitoris
c.   Labia majora
d.   Labia minora

e.   Mons pubis
f.   Perineum
g.   Urethra
h.   Vagina

10. Label the structures of the internal female reproductive organs on the two figures below. Some labels are used more than once. *(22, 23)*

a. Bladder
b. Broad ligament
c. Cervix
d. Fallopian tube
e. Fimbriae

f. Ovary
g. Rectum
h. Uterine fundus
i. Vagina

Student Name_____

11. Match each female reproductive organ with its function or functions (a–r). More than one letter may be used for some organs.

_____ Bartholin's glands (vulvovaginal glands) *(22)*

_____ Cervical mucous membrane *(24)*

_____ Cervix *(24)*

_____ Clitoris *(22)*

_____ Endometrium *(23, 24)*

_____ Fallopian tubes *(24)*

_____ Myometrium *(23)*

_____ Ovaries *(24)*

_____ Rugae *(22)*

_____ Skene's ducts (paraurethral ducts) *(22)*

_____ Urethral meatus *(22)*

_____ Uterus *(22, 23)*

_____ Vagina *(22, 28)*

_____ Vaginal introitus *(22)*

a. Location for implantation of the fertilized ovum and growth of fetus
b. Female organ of sexual intercourse
c. Uterine layer that responds to hormone changes during the menstrual cycle
d. Sensitive erectile body that gives erotic sensations when stimulated
e. Passage for menstrual flow and fetus
f. Folds or ridges of the vaginal mucous membrane
g. Produce vaginal lubrication during sexual arousal
h. Uterine layer in which fertilized ovum implants
i. Site of fertilization and early embryonic development
j. Produce ova (female germ cells) and female hormones
k. Muscular uterine layer to expel fetus at birth
l. Provides an environment favorable to sperm's survival
m. Lubricate urethra and vaginal orifice
n. Division between external and internal female genitals
o. Location for urine to be expelled
p. Narrow, tubular part of the uterus
q. Produces the mucous plug during pregnancy
r. Produces bacteriostatic vaginal lubrication

12. Label each diameter of the pelvic inlet on the figure below and list the normal measurements for each. *(25)*

a. Anteroposterior
b. Transverse
c. Left oblique
d. Right oblique

13. Label each structure of the female breast on the figure below. Some labels may be used on both views. *(26)*

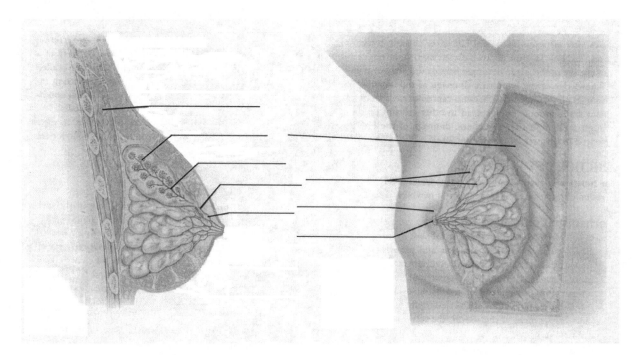

a. Alveolus/alveoli
b. Areola
c. Lactiferous duct

d. Lactiferous sinus
e. Nipple
f. Pectoralis major muscle

14. Match each female breast structure with its function (a–e). *(26)*

_____   Alveolus/alveoli
_____   Areola
_____   Cooper's ligaments
_____   Lactiferous duct
_____   Lactiferous sinus

a. Widened area of a duct that holds milk
b. Glands that secrete milk
c. Carry milk from alveoli to nipple
d. Area of darker skin surrounding nipple
e. Provide support for breast

15. Match each term with its definition (a–e).

_____   Corpus luteum *(26-28)*
_____   Dyspareunia *(22)*
_____   Follicle *(26-28)*
_____   Menarche *(28)*
_____   Ovulation *(26)*

a. Painful sexual intercourse
b. Empty follicle after ovum is released
c. First menstrual period
d. Release of mature ovum
e. Cavity containing a single ovum

Student Name_____

16. State where each of the following female hormones is secreted and its function or functions.

    a. FSH (follicle stimulating hormone) *(26)* _____

         _____

         _____

    b. LH (luteinizing hormone) *(26)* _____

         _____

         _____

    c. Estrogen *(26-28)*_____

         _____

         _____

    d. Progesterone *(26-28)* _____

         _____

         _____

THINKING CRITICALLY

1. Your 11-year-old niece confides to you that she is worried because she had her first menstrual period two months ago but has not had another one. She tells you she learned in school that most girls have periods once each month. What should you tell her?

2. A woman is seeing the nurse practitioner because she has recurrent vaginal infections. She says she douches frequently to "keep herself clean," but that the infections often recur, especially when she needs antibiotics as she is now taking for an ear infection. What advice can the nurse give her?

APPLYING KNOWLEDGE

1. Examine a model of the female pelvis. Identify the following landmarks.
    a. Coccyx
    b. Sacrum
    c. Ischial spine
    d. Symphysis pubis
    e. Ilium
    f. Linea terminalis

2. Identify the following pelvic inlet diameters on a model of the female pelvis. Which diameter of the inlet and outlet is the shortest?

    Inlet:
    a. Anteroposterior
    b. Left and right oblique
    c. Transverse

Cavity:
a.   Interspinous transverse

Outlet:
a.   Anteroposterior
b.   Intertuberous transverse
c.   Anteriorposterior sagittal

REVIEW QUESTIONS

1.   The average female is usually shorter than the average male because: *(19-21)*
     1.   girls have high levels of testosterone during puberty.
     2.   boys begin puberty at an earlier age than girls.
     3.   the growth spurt of girls ends earlier than that of boys.
     4.   onset of puberty stops growth in a girl's height.

2.   A woman can become pregnant even if the male "pulls out" before ejaculation because: *(21)*
     1.   ejaculation occurs before insertion of the penis.
     2.   some semen is released before ejaculation.
     3.   sperm are added to semen after ejaculation.
     4.   semen enters the urethra as soon as the penis is inserted.

3.   A woman comes to the clinic for a yearly checkup pelvic exam. She asks if it is all right for her to use a douche occasionally. The nurse should teach her that douching: *(22)*
     1.   is unnecessary but does no harm if she prefers to do it.
     2.   may hinder her vagina's natural cleansing action.
     3.   adds to the natural cleansing action of her vagina.
     4.   should be avoided because it makes the vagina acidic.

4.   The uterine layer that responds to hormonal changes and receives the fertilized ovum is the: *(23)*
     1.   parametrium.
     2.   myometrium.
     3.   endometrium.

5.   The true pelvis is divided from the false pelvis by the: *(25)*
     1.   obstetric conjugate.
     2.   right and left oblique diameters.
     3.   linea terminalis.
     4.   bi-ischial diameter.

6.   The typical pelvic type for a male is the: *(24-25)*
     1.   android.
     2.   anthropoid.
     3.   gynecoid.
     4.   platypelloid.

7.   The ideal pelvic type for a female is the: *(24-25)*
     1.   android.
     2.   anthropoid.
     3.   gynecoid.
     4.   platypelloid.

Student Name_____

8. Which division of the female pelvis can change slightly to accommodate the fetus during birth? *(26)*
   1. Pelvic inlet
   2. Pelvic cavity
   3. Pelvic outlet

9. Males are generally stronger than females at maturity because: *(21)*
   1. males begin puberty at an earlier age than females.
   2. testosterone promotes growth of a male's muscles.
   3. females start puberty at a later age than males.
   4. high estrogen production promotes bone growth.

10. The function of a male's scrotum is to: *(20)*
    1. regulate the temperature of the testes.
    2. carry sperm from the testes to the penis.
    3. secrete the hormone testosterone.
    4. increase the strength of ejaculation of sperm.

11. The breast structures that secrete milk after childbirth are the: *(26)*
    1. lactiferous ducts.
    2. Montgomery's glands.
    3. alveoli.
    4. nipples.

12. Erection of the penis occurs during sexual stimulation because: *(28)*
    1. smooth muscles attached to the pelvis lift the penis.
    2. blood is trapped within the tissues of the organ.
    3. the testosterone level falls in response to stimulation.
    4. prostate gland secretions cause the organ to stiffen.

13. What is the most appropriate nursing response to the woman who decides she cannot breastfeed because she has small breasts? *(26)*
    1. "Small breasts usually have less milk-secreting tissue, but you could give it a try when the baby arrives."
    2. "Pregnancy hormones will increase most women's breast size enough to feed the average-size infant."
    3. "Small breasts actually have more milk secreting glands than larger breasts; there should be plenty of milk."
    4. "It is the amount of fat in your breasts that determines their size, so your chances of successfully nursing are good."

14. The middle layer of the myometrium has _____ fibers. *(23)*
    1. circular
    2. figure-eight–shaped
    3. longitudinal
    4. oblique

15. The endometrium of the uterus is thinnest at what time? *(23, 26-28)*
    1. Just before ovulation
    2. Between ovulation and menstruation
    3. At the beginning of menstruation
    4. Just after menstruation

CHAPTER 3

Prenatal Development

Answer Key: Textbook page references are provided as a guide for answering these questions. A complete answer key was provided for your instructor.

LEARNING ACTIVITIES

1. Match the terms in the left column with their definitions on the right (a–g).

   _____ Diploid *(30)*
   _____ Gamete *(31)*
   _____ Haploid *(30)*
   _____ Meiosis *(30)*
   _____ Mitosis *(30)*
   _____ Oogenesis *(30)*
   _____ Spermatogenesis *(30)*

   a. Normal number of chromosomes in each mature sperm or ovum
   b. Normal number of chromosomes in nonreproductive cells
   c. Cell division in sex cells
   d. Cell division in non-sex cells to allow growth and replacement of cells
   e. Formation of spermatozoa
   f. Formation of ova
   g. An ovum or spermatozoon

2. a. Spermatogenesis results in the formation of how many sperm from each immature primary spermatocyte? _____ *(30-32)*

   b. Each sperm contains _____ autosomes and either a(n) _____ or a(n) _____ sex chromosome. *(30-32)*

3. a. Oogenesis results in the formation of how many mature ova from each primary oocyte? _____ *(30-32)*

   b. Each ovum contains _____ autosomes and a(n) _____ sex chromosome. *(30-32)*

4. a. An ovum survives about _____ hours after ovulation. *(31-32)*

   b. Sperm survive up to _____ hours after ejaculation. *(31-32)*

5. a. If the ovum is fertilized by a sperm bearing a Y chromosome, the baby will be a _____. *(32-33)*

   b. If the ovum is fertilized by a sperm bearing an X chromosome, the baby will be a _____. *(32-33)*

c. What influence, if any, does the woman have on the sex of the baby that is conceived? *(32-33)*

_____

_____

6. Fertilization usually occurs in the _____. The fertilized ovum usually implants in the _____ section of the _____ uterus. *(33)*

7. Match the terms in the left column with their definitions on the right (a–j).

_____ Amnion *(33)*	a. Inner fetal membrane that envelops the embryo and fetus
_____ Blastocyst *(33)*	b. Outer fetal membrane that envelops the amnion and embryo/fetus
_____ Blastomere *(33)*	
_____ Chorion *(33)*	c. Solid cluster of cells that is approximately the same size as the zygote
_____ Decidua basalis *(33)*	d. Eight-cell stage of prenatal development
_____ Embryo *(36)*	e. Projections on the outer part of fetal side of the placenta that extend into the decidua basalis
_____ Fetus *(36)*	
_____ Morula *(33)*	f. Prenatal development from the second week until the end of the eighth week after fertilization
_____ Chorionic villi *(35-36)*	g. Prenatal development from the ninth week after fertilization until birth
_____ Zygote *(33)*	h. Uterine lining after implantation that gives rise to the maternal side of the placenta
	i. Zygote containing an inner cell mass that will develop into the embryo
	j. Cell formed by union of a sperm and ovum

8. The normal amount of amniotic fluid near the end of pregnancy is about _____ ml. *(33-34)*

9. List the five functions of amniotic fluid. *(34)*

a. _____

b. _____

c. _____

d. _____

e. _____

10. Red blood cells are formed by the _____ for the first six weeks after gestation and then are formed by the _____ and _____, and finally the _____. *(34, 39 [Table 3-1])*

Student Name_____

11. List the tissues that form from each of the three primary germ layers. *(35)*

    Ectoderm

    a. _____

    b. _____

    c. _____

    d. _____

    e. _____

    Mesoderm

    a. _____

    b. _____

    c. _____

    d. _____

    e. _____

    f. _____

    g. _____

    Endoderm

    a. _____

    b. _____

    c. _____

12. List four functions of the placenta. *(36)*

    a. _____

    b. _____

    c. _____

    d. _____

13. Describe the functions of each of the following four placental hormones during pregnancy. *(36, 39)*

    a. Progesterone

    (1) _____

    (2) _____

    (3) _____

    (4) _____

b. Estrogen

   (1) _____

   (2) _____

   (3) _____

   (4) _____

   (5) _____

   (6) _____

c. Human chorionic gonadotropin (hCG)

   _____

d. Human placental lactogen (hPL)

   _____

14. Label each of the structures listed below on the drawing provided. Color areas to indicate high (red), medium (purple), and low (blue) fetal blood oxygenation. Use the lines on the neonate's illustration on the right to explain how fetal shunts close after birth. *(36, 40-41)*

FETUS

NEONATE

a. Ductus venosus
b. Ductus arteriosus
c. Foramen ovale
d. Umbilical arteries
e. Umbilical vein

Student Name_____

15. The umbilical cord should have _____ vein(s) and _____ artery(ies). *(39-40)*

16. State the age when each fetal circulatory structure closes functionally and permanently. *(40)*

	Functionally	*Permanently*
a. Ductus arteriosus	_____	_____
b. Ductus venosus	_____	_____
c. Foramen ovale	_____	_____

17. Match the prenatal ages with their developmental characteristics on the right (a–h).

_____ 3 weeks *(36, 37)*		a. Basic structure of all systems established
_____ 6 weeks *(38)*		b. Possible to monitor fetal status with kick counts
_____ 8 weeks *(36, 37)*		c. Fetal eyes open
_____ 10 weeks *(36)*		d. Fetus now considered full term
_____ 14 weeks *(36)*		e. Tubular heart begins beating; earliest evidence of brain and spinal cord
_____ 20 weeks *(36)*		f. External genitalia may be determined by ultrasound
_____ 28 weeks *(36)*		g. Extremities will move in response to external stimuli
_____ 38 weeks *(36)*		h. Heart has all four chambers

18. a. Describe three things about the umbilical cord. *(39)*

    (1) Where it is inserted into placenta: _____

    (2) Length:_____

    (3) Vessels: _____

    b. Explain the function of Wharton's jelly: *(39)*_____

19. Describe the differences between monozygotic (identical) and dizygotic (fraternal) twins in terms of the following characteristics. *(41-42)*

Characteristic	*Monozygotic*	*Dizygotic*
a. Same sex or different	_____	_____
b. Number of fertilized ova	_____	_____
c. Number of placentas	_____	_____
d. Number of membranes	_____	_____
e. Number of umbilical cords	_____	_____

THINKING CRITICALLY

1. A woman comes to the family planning clinic where you work. She wants to try a natural method of birth control rather than use artificial methods of contraception. What facts must you know about the survival time of the ovum and sperm to help your patient effectively use this form of family planning? See also Chapter 2 for information about the menstrual cycle and Chapter 11 for further information about natural family planning.

2. Your friend is disappointed because she has just had her fourth girl. "My husband wants a son so much," she says. "I feel terrible that I can't have a boy for him." What is an appropriate way to respond to your friend? Role play this situation with a classmate to refine your therapeutic communication skills.

APPLYING KNOWLEDGE

1. Examine a placenta, particularly the insertion of the umbilical cord into the placenta. Identify the following structures.
    a. Amniotic membrane sac
    b. Fetal side
    c. Maternal side
    d. Umbilical vein
    e. Umbilical arteries (How do the arteries look different from the vein?)
    f. Wharton's jelly

2. What are the changes in the percentage of multifetal deliveries during the past 5 years? Are any associated with infertility therapy? What is the average age of mothers who have twins or higher-order multiples? For additional updated information, see the National Center for Health Statistics website: www.cdc.gov/nchs.

REVIEW QUESTIONS

1. Between the second and the eighth week of pregnancy, the developing baby is known as a(n): *(36)*
    1. gamete.
    2. zygote.
    3. embryo.
    4. fetus.

2. Cell division that results in the formation of reproductive cells is known as: *(30)*
    1. mitosis.
    2. meiosis.
    3. fertilization.
    4. dizygotic.

3. How many chromosomes should be contained in the normal sperm or ovum? *(30)*
    1. 23
    2. 46
    3. 69
    4. 92

Student Name_____

4. Which sex chromosome combination results in conception of a male? *(32)*
   1. XX
   2. XY
   3. YY
   4. XO

5. Hereditary or genetic traits are passed from one generation to the next within the: *(32, 34)*
   1. chromosomes.
   2. zygote.
   3. chorionic villi.
   4. somatic cells.

6. After six weeks gestation, fetal red blood cells are manufactured in the: *(34)*
   1. placenta.
   2. liver.
   3. heart.
   4. blastocyst.

7. Which is the outer fetal membrane? *(33)*
   1. Amnion
   2. Chorion
   3. Syncytium
   4. Vernix

8. The primary function of Wharton's jelly is to: *(39)*
   1. allow the best blood flow through the placental vessels.
   2. prevent the fetal membranes from adhering to the fetal skin.
   3. separate maternal blood from fetal blood in the placenta.
   4. carry fetal waste products back to the placenta.

9. Most fetal blood bypasses circulation to the lungs by way of the: *(40)*
   1. ductus venosus.
   2. foramen ovale.
   3. umbilical vein.
   4. umbilical artery.

10. The fetal circulatory structure that carries blood with the lowest oxygen saturation is the: *(39)*
    1. umbilical vein.
    2. umbilical artery.
    3. ductus venosus.
    4. ductus arteriosus.

11. After fertilization, the zygote grows by: *(30)*
    1. meiosis.
    2. mitosis.
    3. oogenesis.
    4. gametogenesis.

12. The foramen ovale closes permanently in about _____ after birth. *(40)*
    1. 1 hour
    2. 1 day
    3. 3 weeks
    4. 3 months

13. The primary purpose of amniotic fluid is to: *(34)*
    1. speed maturation of fetal lungs.
    2. prevent cold stress after birth.
    3. protect the fetus during development.
    4. produce hormones to maintain pregnancy.

14. Fetal waste products are disposed of by the: *(36)*
    1. fetal liver.
    2. placenta.
    3. yolk sac.
    4. endoderm.

15. Inadequate progesterone is likely to result in: *(36, 39)*
    1. release of multiple ova.
    2. spontaneous abortion.
    3. persistence of the corpus luteum.
    4. a mixture of maternal and fetal blood.

16. Fraternal (dizygotic) twins result when: *(41)*
    1. one sperm fertilizes one ovum.
    2. two sperm fertilize one ovum.
    3. one sperm fertilizes two ova
    4. two sperm fertilize two ova.

17. The sex of identical (monozygotic) twins: *(41)*
    1. is always the same.
    2. may or may not be the same.
    3. is always different.
    4. is always one male and one female.

Student Name _____

CHAPTER 4
Prenatal Care and Adaptations to Pregnancy

Answer Key: Textbook page references are provided as a guide for answering these questions. A complete answer key was provided for your instructor.

LEARNING ACTIVITIES

1. Match the terms in the left column with their definitions on the right (a–g).

    _____ Colostrum *(51)*
    _____ Hemorrhoids *(66-67)*
    _____ Mucous plug *(51)*
    _____ Pseudoanemia *(52)*
    _____ Pica *(62)*
    _____ Spider nevi *(54)*
    _____ Trimester *(47)*

    a. Breast secretion that precedes milk; rich in antibodies
    b. Red elevations of skin with lines radiating from center
    c. Varicose veins of rectum and anus
    d. Anemia occurring because red cells increase less than plasma volume
    e. Ingestion of nonfood substances
    f. 13-week period of pregnancy
    g. Seals cervical canal during pregnancy

2. Match the terms describing a woman's obstetrical history with their definitions on the right (a–h).

    _____ Abortion *(47)*
    _____ Gravida *(47)*
    _____ Multigravida *(47)*
    _____ Multipara *(47)*
    _____ Nullipara *(47)*
    _____ Para *(47)*
    _____ Primigravida *(47)*
    _____ Primipara *(47)*

    a. Pregnancy, regardless of duration; pregnant woman
    b. Woman pregnant for the first time
    c. Woman pregnant for the second or subsequent time
    d. Woman who has not delivered a pregnancy of at least 20 weeks gestation
    e. Woman who delivered one or more pregnancies after at least 20 weeks gestation
    f. Woman who has delivered one pregnancy of at least 20 weeks gestation
    g. Woman who has delivered two or more pregnancies of at least 20 weeks gestation
    h. End of pregnancy before 20 weeks of gestation

3. _____ is a formula used to calculate a woman's estimated date of delivery (EDD). Describe how to use this formula. *(45, 48, Box 4-2)*

_____

_____

_____

4. Describe the presumptive signs of pregnancy. *(48-49)*

   a. _____

   b. _____

   c. _____

   d. _____

   e. _____

   f. _____

   g. _____

   These signs and symptoms are called *presumptive* because _____

   _____ .

5. Describe the probable signs of pregnancy. *(49-50)*

   a. _____

   b. _____

   c. _____

   d. _____

   e. _____

   f. _____

   g. _____

   h. _____

   i. _____

   j. _____

   These signs and symptoms are called *probable* because _____

   _____ .

Student Name_____

6. Describe positive signs of pregnancy. At what time during pregnancy can each be detected? *(50-51)*

   a. _____

   _____

   b. _____

   _____

   c. _____

   _____

7. Match the signs and symptoms of pregnancy with their descriptions on the right (a–l).

   _____ Abdominal striae *(49-50)*

   _____ Amenorrhea *(48)*

   _____ Ballottement *(49)*

   _____ Braxton Hicks contractions *(49)*

   _____ Chadwick's sign *(49)*

   _____ Chloasma gravidarum *(48)*

   _____ Funic souffle *(50-51)*

   _____ Goodell's sign *(49)*

   _____ Hegar's sign *(49)*

   _____ Linea nigra *(48-49)*

   _____ Quickening *(49)*

   _____ Uterine souffle *(50-51)*

   a. Bluish color of cervix, vagina, and vulva
   b. Stretch marks
   c. Rebound of fetal part when tapped by examining finger during vaginal examination
   d. Softened lower uterus
   e. Irregular, painless uterine contractions
   f. Blowing sound heard over uterus
   g. Swishing sound of blood circulating through umbilical cord
   h. Cessation of menses
   i. Softened cervix and vagina
   j. Darker pigmented line in midline of abdomen
   k. Movement of fetus felt by mother
   l. Brownish pigmentation of face ("mask of pregnancy")

8. a. _____ is the hormone detected in a positive pregnancy test. *(51)*

   b. Two body fluids used for pregnancy tests are _____ and _____. *(50)*

9. Describe changes that occur in the reproductive organs during pregnancy. *(51)*

   a. Uterus

   Size _____

   Weight _____

   Capacity _____

   b. Cervix _____

   _____

   c. Ovaries _____

   _____

d. Vagina _____

_____

10. Describe changes in other body systems during pregnancy.

a. Breasts: *(51)* _____

_____

_____

b. Respiratory: *(51-52)* _____

_____

_____

c. Cardiovascular: *(52-53)* _____

_____

_____

d. Gastrointestinal: *(53)* _____

_____

_____

e. Urinary: *(53-54)* _____

_____

_____

f. Integumentary and skeletal: *(54)* _____

_____

_____

11. Describe the recommended weight gain if the woman's prepregnancy weight is as follows: *(58)*

a. Normal: _____ to _____ pounds (_____ to _____ kg)

b. Underweight: _____ to _____ pounds (_____ to _____ kg)

c. Overweight: _____ to _____ pounds (_____ to _____ kg)

12. The recommended calorie increase during pregnancy is _____ calories per day. During lactation, the recommended calorie increase is _____ calories per day. *(58, 62-63)*

13. For the following four nutrients, state the amount needed during pregnancy for an adult and list key food sources for each nutrient. Practice how you would actually teach the information to a pregnant woman. Would you add any information when you teach a breastfeeding woman?

a. Protein *(58)* _____

Amount _____

Student Name _____

Sources _____

_____

b. Calcium *(60)* _____

Amount _____

Sources _____

_____

c. Iron *(60-61)* _____

Amount _____

Sources _____

_____

d. Folic acid *(61)* _____

Amount _____

Sources _____

_____

14. Describe how the nurse can help women meet special nutritional needs during pregnancy.

a. Pregnant adolescent *(61-62)* _____

_____

_____

b. Lactose intolerance *(62)* _____

_____

_____

15. List at least three measures the nurse can teach a woman to relieve each common pregnancy discomfort. Note any related abnormal signs or symptoms that should be reported. Practice explaining each relief measure to a pregnant woman. *(66-67)*

a. Nausea _____

_____

b. Increased vaginal discharge _____

_____

c. Fatigue _____

_____

    d. Backache _____

_____

    e. Constipation _____

_____

    f. Varicose veins _____

_____

    g. Hemorrhoids _____

_____

    h. Heartburn _____

_____

    i. Dyspnea and nasal stuffiness _____

_____

    j. Leg cramps _____

_____

    k. Edema of the legs _____

_____

16. Describe the common emotional reactions of a woman during each trimester of pregnancy. *(68-69)*

    a. First _____

_____

    b. Second _____

_____

    c. Third _____

_____

THINKING CRITICALLY

1. Today is June 19. A woman is admitted to the hospital in labor. She tells you that she has not had prenatal care, but that her "due date" is June 26. How many weeks pregnant is the woman if these dates are confirmed with ultrasound?

2. If a woman's expected date of delivery is July 21, using Nagele's rule, what was the first day of her last menstrual period?

3. Have a discussion group that contains both men and women who have had children (they do not have to be nurses or nursing students). Discuss the parts fathers played in any births. Explore the feelings of men in the group about how they view their role in childbirth.

Student Name_____

CASE STUDIES

1. Rosa Garza comes to the clinic for a regular visit at 26 weeks gestation. Her weight gain has been normal (17 pounds), but Rosa tells you that her mother cautioned her not to gain more than 20 pounds or it will be hard to lose the weight after she gives birth. "My mother said that I should not eat salt and that the doctor will probably give me 'water pills' if I gain too much weight." What teaching should you give Rosa about each of her concerns?
    a. Weight gain
    b. Salt (sodium) intake
    c. Diuretics (water pills)

2. Lauren Holt, 30 years old, is pregnant for the first time. She describes herself as a vegetarian, although she says she occasionally eats dairy products and eggs. What nutritional advice can the nurse provide, considering Lauren's pregnancy needs and her food preferences?

APPLYING KNOWLEDGE

1. Each date below represents the first day of a woman's last menstrual period. Use a wheel to calculate the expected date of delivery for each. If you have access to an electronic gestation calculator, use it to make the same calculations. Using today's date, calculate how many weeks the pregnancy has advanced.
    a. January 18
    b. July 13
    c. December 30

2. Use the TPALM system to describe each of the following pregnancy histories.
    a. A woman is pregnant for the fourth time. She had one spontaneous abortion, one child born at 32 weeks gestation who is living, and another living child born at 41 weeks gestation.
    b. A woman is 32 weeks pregnant with her second pregnancy. Her first pregnancy ended with a spontaneous abortion at 8 weeks gestation.

REVIEW QUESTIONS

1. When a woman is 20 weeks pregnant, she is expected to experience: *(49)*
    1. nausea and vomiting.
    2. movement of the fetus.
    3. burning during urination.
    4. yellowish vaginal discharge.

2. A woman is 16 weeks pregnant. During a prenatal visit, she tells the nurse she is worried that her baby might not be normal. How should the nurse interpret this statement? *(68)*
    1. Concerns about doing "everything right" often become the woman's new standard.
    2. It is unusual for women to have these feelings because they do not perceive the baby as "real."
    3. She may have underlying rejection of the fetus that is being expressed in this way.
    4. Her image of the fetus is not realistic, so the nurse should not be concerned.

3. A woman's emotional reaction during the second trimester of pregnancy may be characterized by: *(68)*
    1. fear for her safety during labor.
    2. passive and dependent behavior.
    3. fantasies about the baby's appearance.
    4. dramatic changes in her moods.

4. The purpose of the mucous plug is to: *(51)*
    1. increase the blood supply to the uterus.
    2. block ascent of infection to the uterus.
    3. soften and stretch the cervix.
    4. lubricate the vaginal walls.

5. While lying on the examining table during her prenatal check at 34 weeks, a woman complains of being dizzy and weak. She is pale and her skin is moist. The best nursing intervention to relieve her symptoms is to: *(52)*
    1. have her turn to her side.
    2. tell her to take deep breaths.
    3. help her sit up on the table.
    4. elevate her feet and legs.

6. A woman who is underweight at the beginning of pregnancy should gain how much weight during pregnancy? *(58)*
    1. 15–25 pounds
    2. 25–35 pounds
    3. 28–40 pounds
    4. More than 40 pounds

7. To ensure that a woman has adequate iron intake during pregnancy, it is often recommended that she: *(60-61)*
    1. drink at least one quart of milk per day.
    2. take 30 mg of an iron supplement daily.
    3. eat combinations of meat and grains.
    4. eat 18 mg of iron daily in a variety of foods.

8. What should the nurse teach a pregnant woman about caring for varicose veins in her legs? *(66)*
    1. Apply warm packs to the legs.
    2. Sit down as much as possible.
    3. Stretch the legs while pointing toes.
    4. Elevate the legs when sitting.

9. The primary goal of prenatal care is to assure the woman of: *(44-45)*
    1. labor with a minimum of pain.
    2. the healthiest outcome possible.
    3. improved long-term nutrition.
    4. minimal pregnancy discomforts.

10. A woman who is pregnant with her first baby is called a: *(47)*
    1. multigravida.
    2. para.
    3. nullipara.
    4. primipara.

Student Name_____

11. Which of the following foods are the highest in iron? *(60-61)*
    1. Citrus fruits and melons
    2. Milk, cheese, and other dairy products
    3. Dried beans, potatoes, and legumes
    4. Meat and dark green vegetables

12. Adequate stores of folic acid are needed before conception to: *(61)*
    1. promote adequate expansion of the blood volume.
    2. reduce nausea and vomiting in the first trimester.
    3. limit depletion of calcium from the mother's teeth.
    4. reduce the risk for fetal neural tube defects.

13. The end outcome (goal) for the nursing diagnosis Altered nutrition: less than body requirements related to low prepregnancy weight, is that the patient will: *(60)*
    1. identify recommended nutrient intake during pregnancy.
    2. gain at least 28 pounds by the end of pregnancy.
    3. recognize that good nutrition promotes maternal and fetal health.
    4. state the appropriate calorie increase for pregnancy.

14. The first day of a woman's last menstrual period was September 5. Her estimated date of delivery (EDD) is: *(47-48, Box 4-2)*
    1. April 12.
    2. May 5.
    3. June 12.
    4. July 16.

15. Choose the best intervention to advise a patient to take for relief of constipation during pregnancy. *(68)*
    1. Take a mild laxative no more than three times per week.
    2. Eat several servings of raw fruits and vegetables each day.
    3. Limit fluids to one quart each day, taken between meals.
    4. Wait until the environment is quiet before defecating.

16. The expectant mother is more likely to have leg cramps if she: *(67)*
    1. does not take her iron supplement each day.
    2. increases her fluid intake to eight glasses per day.
    3. stretches each leg while flexing the foot three times each day.
    4. drinks at least 1 to 1.5 quarts of milk each day.

17. A pregnant woman calls the prenatal clinic and says she has a large amount of yellow vaginal discharge. The nurse should instruct the woman to: *(66)*
    1. douche with a commercial vinegar and water solution.
    2. avoid sexual intercourse until the symptoms go away.
    3. wear cotton panties that allow adequate air circulation.
    4. come to the clinic for further evaluation by the physician.

18. The most appropriate teaching for relief of nausea during early pregnancy is to: *(66)*
    1. divide daily food intake into several small meals.
    2. sit upright for 30–60 minutes after meals.
    3. drink at least 8 ounces of liquid with each meal.
    4. eat dry toast or crackers each night before sleep.

19. A pregnant woman is concerned about the "ugly brown spots" on her face. The nurse should teach her that: *(48-49)*
    1. unscented skin lotions may reduce the darkness of the areas.
    2. these are temporary changes due to increased hormones.
    3. she should avoid wearing makeup until the areas fade.
    4. iron supplements sometimes cause temporary skin darkening.

20. It is important to maintain adequate fluid intake during pregnancy primarily to prevent: *(53-54)*
    1. orthostatic hypotension.
    2. edema of the feet and legs.
    3. nausea and vomiting.
    4. urinary tract infection.

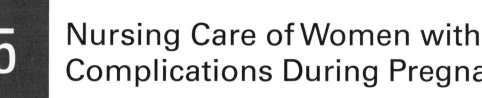

Nursing Care of Women with Complications During Pregnancy

Student Name _____

Answer Key: Textbook page references are provided as a guide for answering these questions. A complete answer key was provided for your instructor.

LEARNING ACTIVITIES

1. Match the terms in the left column with their definitions on the right (a–f).

   _____ Abruptio placentae *(89-90)*
   _____ Ectopic pregnancy *(84-86)*
   _____ Hyperemesis gravidarum *(79, 81-82)*
   _____ Incompetent cervix *(82)*
   _____ Placenta previa *(87, 89)*
   _____ Spontaneous abortion *(82-84)*

   a. Placental attachment in the lower uterus
   b. Premature separation of the normally implanted placenta
   c. Spontaneous loss of a pregnancy before 20 weeks (often called *miscarriage*)
   d. Failure of the cervix to remain closed until the fetus is mature enough to survive outside the uterus
   e. Excessive nausea and vomiting during pregnancy
   f. Development of the fetus outside the uterus

2. List four or more appropriate nursing interventions for the woman with hyperemesis gravidarum. *(79, 81-82)*

   a. _____

   _____

   b. _____

   _____

   c. _____

   _____

   d. _____

   _____

3. Match the types of spontaneous abortion with their descriptions on the right (a–h). *(83)*

    _____ Threatened
    _____ Incomplete
    _____ Inevitable
    _____ Complete
    _____ Missed
    _____ Recurrent
    _____ Therapeutic
    _____ Elective

    a. Bleeding and cramping with cervical dilation but no passage of tissue
    b. Bleeding and cramping with passage of some tissue
    c. Intentional termination of pregnancy for health reasons
    d. Intentional termination of pregnancy for reasons unrelated to health
    e. Passage of all products of conception
    f. Retention of the dead fetus in the uterus
    g. Two or more consecutive spontaneous abortions (also called *habitual abortion*)
    h. Vaginal bleeding without dilation of the cervix or passage of tissue

4. Describe important teaching for a woman after spontaneous abortion for each aspect listed. *(84)*

    a. Bleeding _____

    b. Temperature _____

    c. Iron supplementation _____

    d. Resuming sexual activity _____

    e. Contraception _____

5. An ectopic pregnancy usually occurs in the _____. *(84)*

6. The priority nursing observation related to ectopic pregnancy is for _____. *(86)*

7. Describe each characteristic of gestational trophoblastic disease, also called *hydatidiform mole* or *molar pregnancy*. *(87)*

    a. Bleeding _____

Student Name_____

    b. Uterine size _____

_____

    c. Fetal heart activity _____

_____

    d. Presence of vomiting _____

_____

    e. Blood pressure _____

_____

    f. Human chorionic gonadotropin (hCG) levels _____

_____

    g. Ultrasound appearance _____

_____

    h. Risk for cancer _____

_____

8. Describe the location of each type of placenta previa. *(87)*

    a. Marginal _____

_____

    b. Partial _____

_____

    c. Total _____

_____

9. How does placenta previa compare to abruptio placentae in each of the following characteristics? *(87-90)*

	Placenta Previa	*Abruptio Placentae*
Pain		
Characteristics of bleeding		
Fetal anemia and/or hypoxia		
Consistency of the uterus		
Blood coagulation		
Risk for postpartum hemorrhage		
Risk for postpartum infection		

Student Name _____

10. Using Box 5-1, Danger Signs in Pregnancy, in the textbook, choose the factors that suggest development of gestational hypertension (GH) and the possible cause of each. Which of these suggest that a seizure may occur soon if there is no intervention? *(79, 90)*

_____

_____

_____

_____

_____

_____

_____

_____

11. List six or more factors that increase a woman's risk for development of GH. *(Box 5-4, 91)*

a. _____

b. _____

c. _____

d. _____

e. _____

f. _____

12. Describe each variation of hypertensive disorders of pregnancy. *(Table 5-6, 90-92)*

a. Gestational hypertension _____

_____

b. Preeclampsia _____

_____

c. Eclampsia _____

_____

d. HELLP _____

_____

e. Chronic hypertension _____

_____

f. Preeclampsia with superimposed chronic hypertension _____

_____

13. What blood pressure elevation is significant during pregnancy? *(90)*

_____

14. Describe manifestations of preeclampsia and the cause of each. Note those that suggest severe preeclampsia. *(91)*

    a. Hypertension _____

    _____

    b. Edema _____

    _____

    c. Proteinuria _____

    _____

    d. Central nervous system changes _____

    _____

    e. Visual disturbances _____

    _____

    f. Urine output _____

    _____

    g. Pulmonary edema _____

    _____

    h. Epigastric pain (upper abdominal, over stomach) or nausea _____

    _____

    i. Lab study abnormalities (liver enzymes, coagulation) _____

    _____

15. What is the benefit of activity restriction in treatment of preeclampsia? *(92)*

    _____

16. a. What is the purpose of magnesium sulfate in the treatment of hypertension? *(92-93)*

    _____

    b. What observations are needed for a woman who is receiving magnesium sulfate as treatment for hypertension? *(92-93)*

    _____

Student Name_____

    c.   What drug should be on hand if a woman is receiving magnesium sulfate? *(92-93)*

_____

    d.   What is the desired serum level of magnesium when treating a woman with hypertension? *(92-93)*

_____

17. a.   Rh blood incompatibility can only occur if the mother is Rh _____ and the fetus is Rh _____. *(95-96)*

    b.   The drug given to prevent Rh incompatibility is _____.
(96)

    c.   List four instances in which the drug listed in part (b) is indicated. *(96)*

        (1) _____

        (2) _____

        (3) _____

        (4) _____

18. Which type of diabetes occurs only during pregnancy? *(96, 97)*

_____

19. Describe the test used to screen for gestational diabetes and the normal results. When is screening done? *(97-98)*

_____

_____

_____

20. a.   Why is glucose monitored by blood testing during pregnancy? *(Nursing Care Plan 5-3, 99)*

_____

_____

    b.   What place does urine testing have in diabetes management during pregnancy?

_____ *(Nursing Care Plan 5-3, 99)*

21. The preferred drug used to control the blood glucose during pregnancy is _____ because it _____. *(98)*

22. Describe how insulin requirements change during the course of pregnancy and after birth. *(98)*

_____

_____

23. How may exercise needs differ in the woman who has preexisting diabetes and the woman with gestational diabetes? *(98)*

_____

_____

_____

24. How may the normal changes of pregnancy affect the woman with heart disease? *(102)*

_____

_____

25. How do labor and the postpartum period change the demands on the heart? *(102)*

_____

_____

26. List three reasons why a pregnant woman needs increased iron. *(103)*

    a. _____

    b. _____

    c. _____

27. A woman who is 25 weeks pregnant with her first child has her first prenatal visit. Her initial hemoglobin is 10.8 g/dl. What is the appropriate nursing response to this lab value? *(103)*

_____

_____

_____

28. List foods high in the following nutrients. *(104)*

    a. Iron _____

    _____

    b. Folic acid _____

    _____

    c. Vitamin C _____

    _____

29. a. What types of foods are good to take with an iron supplement and why? *(103)*

    _____

Student Name_____

    b.   What foods or drugs should be avoided at the time an iron supplement is taken and why? *(103)*

_____

_____

30. What are the differences in supplementation of folic acid for routine prevention and actual folic acid deficiency? What two conditions may be prevented by adequate folic acid intake? *(103)*

_____

31. What is the effect of a sickle cell crisis during pregnancy? *(103)*

_____

32. Match each maternal infection with the method to prevent infection of the fetus or newborn on the right (a–f).

_____ Cytomegalovirus *(104)*	a. Deliver infant by cesarean birth if the woman has genital lesions when labor begins
_____ Rubella *(104)*	b. Give immune globulin immediately after birth followed by vaccine
_____ Herpesvirus *(105)*	c. Immunize children to avoid infecting pregnant women; immunize nonimmune woman after birth
_____ Hepatitis B *(105)*	d. Treat culture-positive woman and her infant with penicillin
_____ Toxoplasmosis *(106)*	e. Wash hands and surfaces after handling raw meat, cook meat thoroughly, avoid cat litter
_____ Group B streptococcus *(106-107)*	f. No effective prevention or treatment

33. What are the recommendations to prevent hepatitis B in the newborn? *(105)*

_____

_____

34. List three ways an infant may be infected with human immunodeficiency virus (HIV). *(105-106)*

    a. _____

    b. _____

    c. _____

35. What teaching about the following is appropriate to reduce the spread of HIV? *(106)*

    a. Drug abuse _____

    b. Vaginal intercourse _____

    c. Oral sex _____

36. Why is a pregnant woman more likely to have a urinary tract infection? *(107)*

_____

_____

37. List at least three things the nurse can teach a woman about avoiding a urinary tract infection. *(107)*

   a. _____

   _____

   b. _____

   _____

   c. _____

   _____

38. Describe general approaches to the care of pregnant women related to bioterrorist attacks. *(108)*

   _____

   _____

   _____

39. a.   Describe the manifestations of fetal alcohol syndrome (FAS). *(108-110, Table 5-9)*

   _____

   _____

   b.   What is the current recommendation about alcohol intake during pregnancy? *(108-110, Table 5-9)*

   _____

   _____

40. Match each substance with its potential adverse effects when used during pregnancy or appropriate preventive measures (a–i). *(110)*

   _____ ACE inhibitors

   _____ Cigarette smoking

   _____ Cocaine

   _____ Folic acid antagonists

   _____ Heroin

   _____ Lithium

   _____ Tetracycline

   _____ Vitamin A preparations (isotretinoin [Accutane])

   _____ Warfarin

   a. Abstinence syndrome may develop in woman or infant if drug is stopped suddenly
   b. Associated with congenital heart disease and toxicity to fetal thyroid and kidneys
   c. Causes spontaneous abortion and other serious fetal anomalies
   d. Crosses placenta, possibly causing spontaneous abortion, growth restriction, and Central nervous system and facial defects
   e. Fetal kidney abnormalities, growth restriction, and insufficient amniotic fluid
   f. Infant may be smaller than expected for gestation
   g. Infant may have discolored teeth
   h. Reliable birth control is needed for three months after treatment with this drug
   i. Severe vasoconstriction may cause preterm labor, hypertension with reduced placental circulation, and maternal stroke

41. If a woman needs a potentially teratogenic therapeutic drug during pregnancy, how will the health care provider make a decision about what to prescribe? *(109)*

_____

_____

42. What are the risks to a woman and her infant if she is a victim of abuse? *(109, 111)*

_____

_____

_____

43. List common manifestations of battering. *(111)*

_____

_____

_____

_____

THINKING CRITICALLY

1.   How might anemia affect a woman who has heart disease?

2.   You are helping to care for a woman receiving intravenous magnesium sulfate. You note that her urine output has decreased, and was 20 ml during the past hour. What is the significance of your observation? What is the appropriate action? Why?

3.   If a couple loses a baby at 8 weeks because of spontaneous abortion (miscarriage), how do you think their friends and family are likely to react? What emotional support is appropriate if the woman believes that she should not feel sad because she did not really know the baby yet? How can the nurse help the family cope with this crisis? (These questions can also be enacted by a small group and show both therapeutic and nontherapeutic responses by the nurse. Some group members may be willing to relate personal experiences with a pregnancy loss.)

CASE STUDY

1.   a.   Amy Adams, 28 years old, is pregnant for the fifth time. She has had two spontaneous abortions and one stillborn baby who was born at 35 weeks of gestation. Amy's only living child, Sam, weighed 10 pounds, 3 ounces when born at 36 weeks gestation. Amy had hypertension in her pregnancy with Sam and with her stillborn baby. She is at the clinic for her first prenatal visit at about 20 weeks. An ultrasound accurately determines the gestational age to be 25 weeks. The nurse practitioner determines that Amy began pregnancy about 25 pounds overweight, although her weight gain is normal for 25 weeks. Initial prenatal checks are normal. Identify three or more factors that predispose Amy to complications in this pregnancy. Can any of the risk factors be modified safely? What prenatal assessments may identify these complications early? What danger signals in pregnancy should you teach Amy?

b. Amy's pregnancy progresses normally until 28 weeks gestation. Both the glucose screen (glucose challenge test) and a glucose tolerance test were abnormal, and Amy must take insulin injections twice a day to control her gestational diabetes. What teaching will Amy need for this new problem?

c. Is there a possibility that her diabetes may not be limited to gestational? Why? When is the healthcare provider likely to know that Amy's diabetes is a different type?

d. Amy is 35 weeks pregnant. Her gestational diabetes has been well-controlled, although she has needed higher doses of insulin as pregnancy progressed. She has now developed mild preeclampsia, and her physician admits her to the high-risk pregnancy unit to identify the best therapy for mom and baby. What basic teaching and care are appropriate? How can the nursing staff help Amy and her family cope with the stresses of high-risk pregnancy? What role would an LPN/LVN have in high-risk pregnancy care in your clinical facility?

APPLYING KNOWLEDGE

1. Assist the experienced nurse in assessing each of these reflexes. Will any of these be inaccurate when a woman has epidural analgesia or anesthesia for birth?
   a. Patellar
   b. Biceps
   c. Triceps
   d. Radial

2. Study your hospital's policies and procedures for nursing care related to magnesium sulfate therapy for preeclampsia or eclampsia.

3. Observe the nursing care of a woman who is receiving magnesium sulfate for PIH. What is the reason for each nursing intervention specifically related to magnesium sulfate administration? Did the woman have any of the risk factors for PIH listed in Box 5-4 in the textbook?

4. What foods in your usual diet provide adequate folic acid?

REVIEW QUESTIONS

1. A pregnant woman with type 1 diabetes mellitus asks the nurse why she has needed several increases in her insulin dose during pregnancy. The best answer is that the: *(97)*
   1. pregnancy changes decrease the secretion of insulin from the pancreas.
   2. placenta secretes substances that reduce the effectiveness of insulin.
   3. fetus does not yet secrete insulin and needs more from the mother.
   4. pancreas secretes progressively less insulin as pregnancy progresses.

2. During a seizure of eclampsia, the priority nursing action for a pregnant teen is to: *(93)*
   1. maintain the physical safety to prevent injury.
   2. provide supplemental oxygen by face mask.
   3. insert something between her teeth.
   4. give an anticonvulsant medication.

3. The purpose of the biophysical profile (BPP) is to: *(81, Table 5-1)*
   1. assess the amount of blood incompatibility between the mother and fetus.
   2. determine if the fetal lungs are mature enough to survive extrauterine life.
   3. determine if the placenta is functioning well enough to support fetal life.
   4. identify serious congenital abnormalities during early pregnancy.

Student Name_____

4. If a pregnant woman is not immune to rubella, the expected action is to: *(106)*
    1. limit her contact with other pregnant women.
    2. immunize her early in the postpartum period.
    3. inform her that her baby may have defects.
    4. tell her that there is little risk for problems.

5. Select the most appropriate teaching for the woman who is prone to urinary tract infections. *(107)*
    1. Wipe the perineal area in a front-to-back direction.
    2. Eat a diet high in fiber, iron, and vitamin C.
    3. Eat a diet that includes additional citrus fruits and drinks.
    4. Avoid using added lubricant during sexual intercourse.

6. If a woman has cardiac disease, the main risks to the fetus are related to: *(102)*
    1. poor oxygenation.
    2. preterm birth.
    3. maternal infection.
    4. congenital anomalies.

7. Which of the following fetal or neonatal problems should the nurse anticipate if a woman has persistent hyperemesis gravidarum? *(79-80)*
    1. Multiple vitamin and mineral deficiencies
    2. Poor attachment behaviors at birth
    3. Smaller than expected birth weight
    4. Intrauterine infection or neonatal sepsis

8. Choose the maternal sign or symptom that is most characteristic of hypovolemic shock associated with blood loss in a pregnant woman. *(86, Box 5-2)*
    1. Oral temperature below 36.1° C (97° F)
    2. Abnormal uterine contractions
    3. Urine output of 100 ml/hour
    4. Weak pulse that increases in rate

9. Choose the assessment that should be promptly reported to the physician when a woman is being observed in the emergency room for possible ectopic pregnancy. *(86, Box 5-2)*
    1. Pulse of 88 and blood pressure of 124/66
    2. Light vaginal bleeding without cramping
    3. Oral temperature of 37.3° C (99.2° F)
    4. Fall in urine output to 20 ml/hour

10. The nurse should emphasize the importance of long-term follow-up care for the woman who has a hydatidiform mole to detect the occurrence of: *(87)*
    1. recurrent pregnancy.
    2. choriocarcinoma.
    3. hypertension.
    4. continued bleeding.

11. A significant difference between the signs of abruptio placentae and those of placenta previa is that abruptio placentae involves: *(88-90)*
    1. bleeding.
    2. infection.
    3. vomiting.
    4. pain.

12. A woman is admitted to the hospital with painless vaginal bleeding at 36 weeks of gestation. Which test should the nurse expect? *(80)*
    1. X-ray
    2. Ultrasound
    3. Vaginal exam
    4. Alpha-fetoprotein

13. The cause of preeclampsia is: *(90)*
    1. poor nutrition.
    2. excess weight gain.
    3. multiple fetuses.
    4. unknown.

14. A woman who is hospitalized with severe preeclampsia should be closely observed for the onset of: *(91-92)*
    1. seizures.
    2. proteinuria.
    3. hypotension.
    4. edema.

15. The drug used to reverse magnesium toxicity is: *(92)*
    1. ferrous oxide.
    2. calcium gluconate.
    3. lactated Ringer's.
    4. magnesium chloride.

16. Teaching of the woman who has herpesvirus infection should include: *(105)*
    1. antibiotic treatment of the baby after birth.
    2. the possibility of birth by cesarean delivery.
    3. the minor effects of herpes infection on a newborn.
    4. that immunity is permanent after initial infection.

17. The physician wants to do a group B streptococcus culture when a woman has a prenatal visit at 35 weeks gestation. The woman asks the nurse why the physician is just now concerned about this problem. The best explanation by the nurse is that: *(106)*
    1. determining if she is positive for the organism reduces the risk for spreading it by unwashed or inadequately washed hands.
    2. the woman can carry the organism without knowing it, possibly causing serious infections to her or the newborn.
    3. late-pregnancy infection causes significant delay in fetal lung maturation, causing problems similar to those of prematurity.
    4. tissues of the vaginal and perineal area are more susceptible to tearing at birth when infection occurs during late pregnancy.

18. The nurse should expect to teach the pregnant woman with gestational diabetes to monitor her glucose by: *(Nursing Care Plan 5-3, 98-100)*
    1. assessing blood levels several times a day.
    2. determining levels in the urine twice a day.
    3. recording monthly glycosylated hemoglobin levels.
    4. keeping a written record of hypoglycemic symptoms.

Student Name_____

19. Teaching for the pregnant woman who was newly diagnosed with tuberculosis should include: *(98, Nursing Care Plan 5-3, 106-107)*
    1. increasing fluid intake to 2 quarts each day.
    2. the expectation that birth will require a cesarean delivery.
    3. the importance of taking the entire course of medication.
    4. avoiding contact with family members until all medication is taken.

20. To improve circulation to the placenta in a pregnant woman who has been in a serious car accident, the nurse should: *(112)*
    1. place the woman in a slight head-down position on a horizontal surface.
    2. give all intravenous fluids by pump to reduce fluid overload on her heart.
    3. take vital signs every 15 minutes if her condition is not stable.
    4. place a small pillow under one hip if she must lie on her back.

6 Nursing Care of Mother and Infant During Labor and Birth

Answer Key: Textbook page references are provided as a guide for answering these questions. A complete answer key was provided for your instructor.

LEARNING ACTIVITIES

1. List the "4 Ps" of the birth process. *(119-125)*

   a. _____

   b. _____

   c. _____

   d. _____

2. The two powers of labor are: *(119-122)*

   a. _____

   b. _____

3. a. The amount of cervical dilation is expressed in _____. *(120-121; Fig 6-3)*

   b. Cervical effacement is expressed as _____. *(120-121; Fig 6-3)*

4. The nurse should promptly report contraction durations longer than _____ seconds or intervals shorter than _____ seconds and a frequency closer than every _____ minutes. Why? *(120-122)*

   _____

   _____

5. State two reasons why the sutures and fontanels of the fetal head are important in the birth process. *(122)*

   a. _____

   _____

   b. _____

   _____

6. The abbreviations below describe fetal presentation and position. Spell out each and identify the one describing a breech presentation, the one describing a face presentation, and the one that is the most common of those listed. Identify the fetal presentation and position that often causes "back labor" during birth. *(124-126, Box 6-1; Figure 6-8)*

   a. RSA _____

   b. LMT _____

   c. ROA _____

   d. LOP _____

7. The key difference between true labor and false labor is _____
   _____. *(130-131, Table 6-2)*

8. List the three phases of the first stage of labor. Describe cervical changes and the approximate duration of each phase. *(140-141, Table 6-3)*

   a. _____

   _____

   b. _____

   _____

   c. _____

   _____

9. The fourth stage of labor is _____

   _____

   _____ . *(141, Table 6-3; 148)*

10. Describe typical maternal behaviors or occurrences during each stage and phase of labor. *(140-141)*

   a. First stage

      Latent phase _____

      _____

      Active phase _____

      _____

      Transition phase _____

      _____

   b. Second stage _____

      _____

Student Name_____

   c.   Third stage _____

       _____

   d.   Fourth stage _____

       _____

11. Describe characteristics of the normal fetal heart rate at term. *(132, 134-136, Box 6-3)*

     Rate _____ (lower limit) to _____ (upper limit)

     Other characteristics _____

     _____

12. Describe three characteristics of abnormal amniotic fluid. *(136)*

     _____

     _____

     _____

13. Describe the assessments in the following categories that the nurse should promptly report when caring for a laboring woman. *(136, 137, Box 6-3)*

   a.   Temperature _____

   b.   Blood pressure _____

   c.   Fetal heart rate _____

14. What is the significance of the following patterns on the electronic fetal monitor? Include the nursing response to each, as appropriate. *(133-136)*

   a.   Variability _____

       _____

   b.   Accelerations _____

       _____

   c.   Early decelerations _____

       _____

   d.   Variable decelerations _____

       _____

   e.   Late decelerations _____

       _____

THINKING CRITICALLY

1. The following chart shows a typical status report often used in intrapartum units. Interpret the data about each woman's labor by answering the questions below.

Name	Gravida	Para	Gest	Dil	Eff	Sta	FHR
Amy	2	0	36	1–2	50%	−2	160
Becky	4	3	42	6	80%	−1	115
Cathy	1	0	40	3–4	90%	0	144
Deanna	3	1	39	C	C	+2	132

    a. Which client(s) is/are at full-term gestation?
    b. Which fetus(es) is/are engaged?
    c. Who is likely to deliver soonest? Why?

2. Calculate the 1- and 5-minute Apgar scores on the following infants. Describe nursing actions that relate to these scores. *(143, Table 6-4, 150)*

Sign	Baby boy		Twin A (girl)		Twin B (girl)	
	1 min	*5 min*	*1 min*	*5 min*	*1 min*	*5 min*
Heart rate	125	155	88	130	110	90
Respiratory effort	Strong cry	Reacts spontaneously	Weak cry	Strong cry	Weak cry	Weak cry
Muscle tone	Flexed body	Maintains flexion	Limp	Sluggish movement	Sluggish movement	Sluggish movement
Reflex irritability	Cries and flexes body when suctioned	Cries when suctioned or stimulated	Minimal response to suction	Cries when suctioned or stimulated	Active movement when suctioned	Minimal response to suction
Color	Pink body, blue hands and feet	Pink body, blue hands and feet	Pale	Pink body, blue hands and feet	Pink body, blue hands and feet	Blue body and extremities
TOTAL SCORES						

3. What is the primary reason for observing the maternal bladder closely immediately after birth?

CASE STUDIES

1. A nurse working in a prenatal clinic must teach a woman who does not speak the same language when to go to the hospital. The woman is having her third baby, the first in the United States. Her first labor lasted 18 hours and her second labor lasted 6 hours. What should the nurse teach this woman? Give a rationale for each part of your teaching.

2. A woman is in labor with her first baby. Her cervix is 7 cm dilated, and the fetal station is +1. Formulate appropriate nursing interventions for the nursing diagnosis Acute pain related to labor process and exertion of labor.

Student Name_____

APPLYING KNOWLEDGE

1. Use a model of a pelvis and fetal head to place the head in each of the following positions. Move the head through each mechanism of labor for each of the positions.

   a. ROA   d. LOA   f. LOP

   b. ROT   e. LOT   g. OA

   c. ROP

2. During your clinical experience, note how different fetal presentations or positions affect the woman's comfort during labor. Note if there is an apparent effect on the length of labor.

3. Palpate the uterine contractions of women in labor and classify them as mild, moderate, or firm intensity. Confirm your observations with an experienced intrapartum nurse.

4. Observe the labor of a woman having a vaginal birth after cesarean (VBAC) for the following factors related to her experience.
   a. number of previous cesarean and vaginal births
   b. reason for previous cesarean birth
   c. the woman's desire to have this baby vaginally
   d. maternal behaviors during labor
   e. support of her partner
   f. her apparent feelings after birth, whether it was VBAC or a repeat cesarean

5. Examine electronic fetal monitor strips to identify the following features:
   a. information that the monitor automatically prints on the strip or the screen
   b. interface with computer device, if any
   c. differences in appearance between those obtained with external devices and those from internal devices
   d. presence or absence of variability, rate accelerations, and deceleration patterns
   e. nursing and medical responses to abnormal patterns; fetal response to interventions
   f. outcome of birth, including Apgar scores of the infant

6. Locate the "precip tray" (which may have a different name) in your clinical facility. What are the contents of this tray?

REVIEW QUESTIONS

1. During labor, a baseline fetal heart rate of 125 bpm should be interpreted as: *(133-136)*
   1. normal for a term fetus.
   2. abnormal if the fetus is preterm.
   3. high normal when in labor.
   4. a slow baseline fetal heart rate.

2. When assessing the duration of labor contractions, the nurse should time from the: *(120-121)*
   1. beginning of one contraction to the end of the same contraction.
   2. end of one contraction to the beginning of the next.
   3. beginning of one contraction to the beginning of the next.
   4. peak of one contraction to the end of the contraction.

3. During normal labor, contractions characteristically become: *(Table 6-2, 131; Table 6-3, 140-141)*
   1. more frequent and of shorter duration.
   2. more frequent and of longer duration.
   3. less frequent and of shorter duration.
   4. less frequent and of longer duration.

4. When the fetus is in a cephalic presentation, the amniotic fluid is expected to be: *(136)*
   1. cloudy.
   2. clear.
   3. green.
   4. yellow.

5. The thinning of the cervix during labor is called: *(120)*
   1. dilation.
   2. effacement.
   3. station.
   4. presentation.

6. How should the nurse interpret the abbreviation *ROP*? *(124-125)*
   1. The fetal sacrum is in the mother's right posterior pelvis.
   2. The fetal pelvis is in the mother's right occipital pelvis.
   3. The fetal occiput is in the mother's right posterior pelvis.
   4. The right fetal occiput is in the mother's posterior pelvis.

7. The labor phase when the woman often feels anxious, restless, and seems to lose control is: *(140-141)*
   1. latent.
   2. active.
   3. transition.
   4. placental.

8. Thirty minutes after birth, the nurse assesses the woman's uterine fundus. It is firm, above her umbilicus, and deviated to the right side. The appropriate nursing action is to: *(148)*
   1. massage the uterus.
   2. assist her to urinate.
   3. provide mild analgesia.
   4. restrict oral intake.

9. Choose the abbreviation that describes the fetus in a breech presentation. *(124-125)*
   1. LSA
   2. OA
   3. ROA
   4. LMT

10. Which sign or symptom normally occurs shortly before labor begins? *(125)*
    1. An urge to push or bear down
    2. Increased clear vaginal discharge
    3. Moderate amount of vaginal bleeding
    4. Sudden weight gain of 3–5 pounds

Student Name_____

11. Fetal descent during labor is measured in relation to the mother's: *(128)*
    1. posterior perineum.
    2. sacral promontory.
    3. ischial spines.
    4. uterine fundus.

12. When the placenta is delivered with the fetal side presenting, the mechanism is called: *(141, 143, 144)*
    1. Duncan.
    2. Lamaze.
    3. VBAC.
    4. Schultz.

13. During the latent phase of labor, the nurse should expect the woman's behavior to be: *(140)*
    1. sleepy, except during contractions.
    2. mildly anxious, coping with contractions.
    3. quiet, concentrating on each contraction.
    4. frustrated, losing control with contractions.

14. A woman's membranes rupture during labor. The nurse notes that the fluid is yellowish and cloudy. The priority nursing response related to this assessment is to: *(136)*
    1. remove wet underpads and replace them with dry ones.
    2. perform a vaginal examination to assess labor progress.
    3. reassure the woman that membrane rupture is expected.
    4. assess the woman's temperature and the fetal heart rate.

15. The nurse should learn to evaluate labor progress by methods other than vaginal examination, primarily because vaginal examination: *(137)*
    1. worsens the mother's discomfort.
    2. increases the risk for infection.
    3. reduces fetal heart rate variability.
    4. delays normal progression of labor.

16. Of the following, which is the priority for nursing care during the second stage of labor? *(129, 138, 140-141)*
    1. Observe the woman's perineum.
    2. Encourage pushing with contractions.
    3. Evaluate labor coping skills.
    4. Administer ordered analgesia.

17. Which maternal position should be avoided during labor? *(136)*
    1. Sitting
    2. Walking
    3. Side-lying
    4. Supine

18. The woman having a vaginal birth after cesarean (VBAC) should be observed during labor particularly for signs of: *(142)*
    1. labor progression.
    2. uterine rupture.
    3. perineal pressure.
    4. excessive anxiety.

19. Which nursing assessment finding should be promptly reported to the physician or nurse-midwife? *(120, 136)*
    1. Clear amniotic fluid containing white flecks
    2. Fetal heart rate of 145 bpm with variability
    3. Vaginal discharge of mucus with dark blood
    4. Contraction intervals shorter than 2 minutes

20. The priority nursing observation during the fourth stage is for: *(141, 148)*
    1. vaginal bleeding.
    2. perineal bulging.
    3. uterine infection.
    4. parent-infant bonding.

21. When assessing labor contractions, the nurse notes that the contracting uterus can be slightly indented with the fingertips when contractions are at their peak. Contraction intensity should be recorded as: *(121)*
    1. mild.
    2. moderate.
    3. firm.
    4. latent.

22. A woman phones the birth center and says, "I think my water broke and my baby is due, but I'm not having any contractions." The most appropriate nursing response is to tell her that: *(126, 128-129)*
    1. labor should begin within a few hours at most.
    2. urine leakage may be confused with ruptured membranes.
    3. she should come to the birth center for evaluation.
    4. there is no concern unless the fluid is bloody.

23. Amniotic fluid usually turns Nitrazine paper: *(136)*
    1. yellow.
    2. green.
    3. dark blue.
    4. purple.

24. The nurse notes a pattern of variable decelerations on the electronic fetal monitor strip. The initial nursing response should be to: *(135-136)*
    1. reassure the woman that the pattern is expected.
    2. change the laboring woman's position.
    3. increase the rate of the nonadditive IV fluid.
    4. notify the physician of the abnormal pattern.

Student Name_____

25. The primary means to identify hemorrhage after vaginal birth is to: *(148)*
    1. assess the vital signs frequently.
    2. observe the uterine fundus and lochia.
    3. keep an ice pack on the perineum.
    4. have the woman urinate every 2 hours.

26. The term infant may be placed in skin-to-skin contact with the mother immediately after birth primarily for the purpose of: *(Skill 6-1, 129; 149)*
    1. breastfeeding while the baby is alert.
    2. maintaining the infant's temperature.
    3. promoting early parent-infant attachment.
    4. stimulating expulsion of the placenta.

CROSSWORD PUZZLE

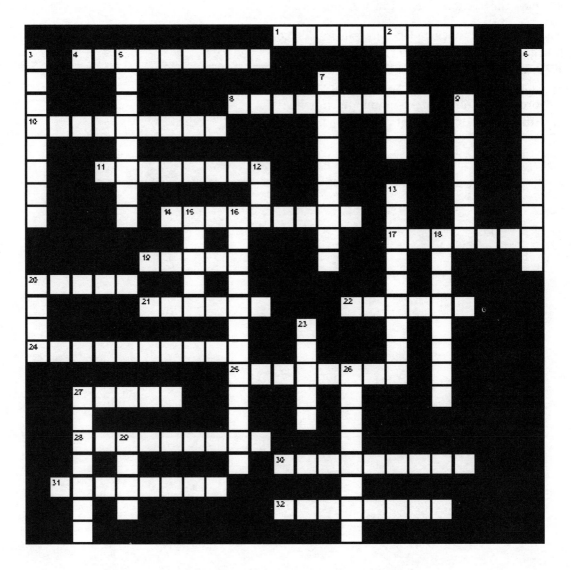

Student Name_____

Across

1. Strength of labor contractions *(121)*
4. Time from the beginning of one contraction until the beginning of the next *(120)*
8. Pivoting of fetal head under the mother's symphysis pubis during labor *(128)*
10. Period of increasing strength of a labor contraction *(120)*
11. Fetal rotation as the head turns within the mother's pelvis *(127-128)*
14. Middle part of the true pelvis *(122)*
17. Level of the fetal presenting part in relation to the ischial spines in the pelvis *(126)*
19. Upper flaring part of the mother's pelvis *(122)*
20. Stage of labor from the baby's birth until delivery of the placenta *(141, 148)*
21. Part of the true pelvis that is nearest the perineum *(122)*
22. Fetal substance that may normally be found in amniotic fluid *(136)*
24. Thinning of the cervix *(120)*
25. Fontanel that has four suture lines leading to it *(122-123)*
27. Stage of labor from its onset to complete cervical dilation *(140-141)*
28. Birth of the fetal shoulders and body *(127-128)*
30. Period of decreasing strength of a labor contraction *(120)*
31. Opening of the cervix *(120)*
32. Length of a labor contraction from its beginning to its end *(120-121)*

Down

2. Maternal pushing occurs during this stage of labor *(140-141)*
3. Orientation of a fixed point on the fetus to the mother's pelvis *(124)*
5. Fetal rotation as the head turns to face one of the mother's thighs *(127-128)*
6. Descent of the fetal presenting part to a zero station or lower *(127-128)*
7. Amniotic fluid may be cloudy if this condition is present *(136)*
9. Downward progress of fetal presenting part *(126)*
12. Orientation of the fetus in relation to the mother's spine *(122)*
13. Fontanel that has three suture lines leading into it *(122-123)*
15. Upper part of the true pelvis *(122)*
16. Fetal part that enters pelvis first *(123)*
18. Fetal flexion or extension *(122-123)*
20. Lower portion of pelvis *(122)*
23. Characteristic of normal amniotic fluid *(136)*
26. Relaxation period between two labor contractions *(122)*
27. Bending of the fetal head toward the chest *(123-124, 128)*
29. Period of greatest strength of a labor contraction *(120)*

CHAPTER 7

Student Name _____

Nursing Management of Pain During Labor and Birth

Answer Key: Textbook page references are provided as a guide for answering these questions. A complete answer key was provided for your instructor.

LEARNING ACTIVITIES

1. Match the terms in the left column with their definitions on the right (a–e).

    _____ Effleurage *(157)*
    _____ Endorphins *(158)*
    _____ Focal point *(157, 160)*
    _____ Pain threshold *(156)*
    _____ Pain tolerance *(156)*

    a. Least amount of stimulation that a person perceives as painful
    b. Maximum amount of pain one is willing to bear
    c. Stroking of the abdomen, thighs, or other body parts
    d. Intense concentration on an object
    e. Internal substances similar to morphine

2. List four physical factors that cause pain during labor. *(158)*

    a. _____

    b. _____

    c. _____

    d. _____

3. How do each of these physical factors influence a woman's pain during labor? *(158)*

    a. Cervical readiness _____

    _____

    b. Pelvic size and shape _____

    _____

    c. Labor intensity _____

    _____

    d. Maternal fatigue _____

    _____

e.   Fetal presentation and position _____

_____

4.   How does a woman's anxiety or fear relate to labor pain? *(156, 159)*

_____

_____

5.   How can each aspect of prenatal classes help a woman in labor? *(154-157, Box 7-1)*

a.   Education about expected changes _____

_____

b.   Conditioning exercise _____

_____

c.   Identify classes offered at your clinical facility, who teaches them, and the classes that continue after birth. _____

_____

6.   List three reasons why it is useful for any laboring woman to know nonpharmacologic pain control methods. *(159)*

a.   _____

b.   _____

c.   _____

7.   a.   Explain why promoting a woman's relaxation during labor is essential to any type of pain management. *(157, 159)*

_____

_____

b.   Describe at least four ways to help the laboring woman relax. *(159)*

_____

_____

_____

_____

8.   What nursing care may help a woman cope with the following problems during labor? *(161-162, Box 7-2)*

a.   Hyperventilation _____

_____

Student Name _____

    b. Urge to push before complete cervical dilation _____

    _____

9. Explain the differences between these anesthesia professionals. *(162)*

    a. Anesthesiologist _____

    _____

    b. Certified registered nurse anesthetist (CRNA) _____

    _____

10. Explain why it is usually best to avoid opioid narcotic analgesics if birth is anticipated within 1 hour of administration. *(163, Table 7-1)*

    _____

    _____

11. What is the purpose of naloxone (Narcan)? What is an important nursing observation of the newborn related to use of this drug? *(163)*

    _____

    _____

12. For each type of regional anesthetic listed below, describe (a) how it is administered, (b) the location of its pain relief, (c) its major side effects, and (d) medical and nursing measures related to its use.

    Local infiltration (164-165)

    a. _____

    _____

    b. _____

    _____

    c. _____

    _____

    d. _____

    _____

Pudendal block (164-165)

a. _____

_____

b. _____

_____

c. _____

_____

d. _____

_____

Epidural block (165-166)

a. _____

_____

b. _____

_____

c. _____

_____

d. _____

_____

Subarachnoid block (167)

a. _____

_____

b. _____

_____

c. _____

_____

d. _____

_____

13. An anesthesiologist often gives a test dose of the anesthetic agent when starting an epidural block to
identify _____.

The expected reaction to the test dose is _____. *(165)*

Student Name _____

14. The woman who plans to have epidural anesthesia during labor and birth should be particularly questioned about allergy to _____. Why? _____

_____ *(164, 166)*

15. What is potentially the most life-threatening complication of general anesthesia for the mother? What is done to reduce the risk? *(164, 167, Table 7-2)*

_____

_____

16. A woman receives epidural morphine sulfate (Astramorph) after a cesarean birth. What should the nurse expect to assess related to this drug and for how long? *(171)*

_____

THINKING CRITICALLY

1. Why do you think general anesthesia is seldom used for vaginal delivery in the United States or Canada?

2. A woman who is 2 hours postpartum after an uncomplicated birth wants to go to the bathroom to urinate. She had an epidural block for pain relief during labor and the medication and catheter for the block were removed immediately after birth. The infant has been nursing at intervals and the mother has eaten a light meal.
   a. Should you allow her to use the bathroom or have her use a bedpan? Explain the reason for your choice.
   b. If you allow her to walk to the bathroom, describe what you should do to ensure her safety.

3. Discuss interventions of health professionals for women during labor with your classmates. What did you observe that reduced the woman's anxiety and pain? What increased anxiety and pain and was it possible to change these outcomes?

CASE STUDIES

1. a. Jill Sims is a primigravida in labor at 4 cm cervical dilation. She is using breathing techniques she learned in prepared childbirth classes. Jill is breathing rapidly throughout each contraction. She complains of stiff fingers and numbness around her mouth. What is the probable cause of Jill's symptoms? What is an appropriate nursing measure to help correct her problem?
   b. Jill is now 5–6 cm dilated and requests an epidural block. Is this an appropriate time during labor to give an epidural block? If so, what nursing observations are most important before and after the block is begun?
   c. What nursing measures are appropriate during second stage labor?

2. You are working with a laboring woman and note that she is holding her body stiffly and gripping the bed rails tightly during each contraction. What nursing interventions are appropriate in each of the following areas? (This activity can be used to demonstrate the techniques for a clinical conference. If so, suggest additional techniques.)
   a. Relaxation techniques
   b. Adjusting the environment
   c. Assisting her with breathing techniques

APPLYING KNOWLEDGE

1. When you are in the hospital, look at trays used to administer various anesthetics. Identify the following components in the trays.
   a. Pudendal block tray: trumpet
   b. Epidural block tray: Touhy or other needle used to insert into the epidural space, epidural catheter, and sizes of the needles and catheter
   c. Subarachnoid (spinal) block tray: spinal needle (note any size difference from the epidural needle)

2. Identify professionals in your hospital who administer obstetrical anesthesia. Are they limited to administration of specific types of anesthesia? Is one present 24 hours a day? Do obstetricians give epidural blocks?

3. Look at the contents of emergency carts for women and newborns. Who usually handles emergency care of newborns who are in distress? Do they hold certification from the American Heart Association and American Academy of Pediatrics in neonatal resuscitation (NRP)? Which professionals are present at uncomplicated births or cesarean births to care for the infant?

4. What is the most common anesthesia for vaginal birth in your hospital? For cesarean birth?

5. Observe a childbirth education class.

6. Observe a laboring woman using childbirth preparation techniques. Who is her support person? How is the support person helping her use these techniques? How can you help her?

REVIEW QUESTIONS

1. According to the gate control theory, which technique should be most helpful in interrupting transmission of labor pain to the brain? *(159)*
   1. Rapid, shallow breathing
   2. Application of heat
   3. Focusing on a point in the room
   4. Deep, cleansing breaths

2. Choose the best method during the admission process to help relieve general anxiety for a woman having her first baby who has not attended prepared childbirth classes. *(162)*
   1. Assure her that she will be given pain medication any time she needs it.
   2. Determine her reasons for not attending the classes offered in the hospital.
   3. Have her take deep breaths to relax all muscles before doing any admission assessments.
   4. Give simple explanations about her environment and what to expect during labor.

3. Butorphanol differs from meperidine in that butorphanol: *(163)*
   1. should not be used if a woman is dependent on heroin.
   2. causes greater respiratory depression in the newborn.
   3. better reduces the pain of late labor.
   4. cannot be reversed with naloxone.

4. The newborn of a woman who receives narcotic analgesics during labor should be observed primarily for: *(163, 171)*
   1. convulsions.
   2. slow respirations.
   3. excess activity.
   4. constipation.

Student Name_____

5. A woman (gravida 2, para 1) plans an epidural block for labor and birth. Which factor in her history is most significant in terms of her planned anesthetic? *(164-165)*
   1. Mild hypertension during first pregnancy
   2. Light meal 4 hours before labor began
   3. Forceps delivery during first birth
   4. Adverse reaction to dental anesthetic

6. An advantage of an epidural block is that it: *(164-166)*
   1. reduces pain for both labor and birth.
   2. has no fetal or maternal risks.
   3. supports normal blood pressure.
   4. enhances the woman's urge to push.

7. Immediately after birth, nursing care for the woman who had subarachnoid block anesthesia for a repeat cesarean birth should include: *(164, 167)*
   1. ambulating within 2 hours of birth.
   2. keeping her back curved outward.
   3. assessing for return of sensation.
   4. keeping her flat in bed for 8 hours.

8. A blood patch may be done to relieve: *(167)*
   1. low blood pressure.
   2. respiratory depression.
   3. postspinal headache.
   4. prolonged numbness.

9. The nurse should observe the woman who received epidural opioid narcotics for: *(171)*
   1. late respiratory depression.
   2. nausea and vomiting.
   3. unstable blood pressure.
   4. persistent headache.

10. During general anesthesia, cricoid pressure is applied to: *(164, 167)*
    1. reduce stomach acid secretion.
    2. avoid aspiration of gastric contents.
    3. prevent excessive blood loss.
    4. limit musculoskeletal injuries.

11. A woman asks if she should take prepared childbirth classes. The best response of the nurse is to tell her that classes will: *(159)*
    1. allow her to avoid pain medications during labor.
    2. be required if her partner wants to be with her.
    3. provide methods to help her cope with labor.
    4. reduce the likelihood that complications will occur.

12. The prepared childbirth technique that is most likely to relieve back pain during labor is: *(160)*
    1. effleurage.
    2. sacral pressure.
    3. thermal stimulation.
    4. patterned breathing.

13. A woman is using prepared childbirth breathing techniques and complains of dizziness and tingling. The nurse should: *(161)*
    1. have her breathe more rapidly with contractions.
    2. ask her if she feels an urge to push or bear down.
    3. tell her to exhale slowly into her cupped hands.
    4. reassure her that these sensations are normal.

14. Immediately after an epidural block is begun, the woman may be positioned: *(162, 165)*
    1. flat on her back, with no pillow.
    2. sitting upright with her legs over the side of the bed.
    3. with a small roll under her hip.
    4. in a modified Trendelenburg position.

15. Two hours after a vaginal birth with an epidural anesthesia, the nurse determines that the woman's bladder is full. The most appropriate initial nursing action is to: *(164, 166)*
    1. help her walk to the bathroom if movement and sensation have returned.
    2. ask her how full her bladder feels before allowing her to walk to the bathroom.
    3. insert an indwelling (Foley) catheter until the woman is at least 8 hours postpartum.
    4. take no action unless the woman says her full bladder makes her uncomfortable.

16. The most effective way to identify adequate maternal oxygenation after epidural narcotic for cesarean birth is to: *(170, 171)*
    1. take the blood pressure regularly.
    2. observe for cyanosis or restlessness.
    3. maintain a side-lying position.
    4. observe pulse-oximeter readings.

CHAPTER 8

Nursing Care of Women with Complications During Labor and Birth

Answer Key: Textbook page references are provided as a guide for answering these questions. A complete answer key was provided for your instructor.

LEARNING ACTIVITIES

1. Match the terms in the left column with their definitions on the right (a–h).

   _____ Amniotomy *(173)*

   _____ Cephalopelvic disproportion *(180, 184)*

   _____ Chignon *(179)*

   _____ Chorioamnionitis *(192-193)*

   _____ Dystocia *(184, 187, 191)*

   _____ Hydramnios *(174, 184, 186)*

   _____ Laminaria *(175)*

   _____ Macrosomia *(187)*

   a. Infection of the amniotic sac
   b. Excessive amniotic fluid
   c. Substance that swells within the cervix, dilating it slightly
   d. Circular swelling on the neonate's head caused by vacuum extractor
   e. Large body size
   f. Artificial rupture of the amniotic sac
   g. Inability of the fetus to fit through the pelvis
   h. Difficult labor

2. Describe three potential complications of amniotomy and the nursing assessments that should be done and recorded for each. *(173-174)*

   a. _____

   _____

   b. _____

   _____

   c. _____

   _____

3. Distinguish between labor *induction* and labor *augmentation.* *(174-176)*

   _____

   _____

4. Identify each drug or class of drugs from the following descriptions of their main purpose. Give examples of specific drugs for c and d.

   a. Soften the cervix *(175)* _____

   _____

   b. Stimulate labor contractions *(175)* _____

   _____

   c. Inhibit uterine contractions *(175, 193)* _____

   _____

   d. Speed fetal lung maturation *(193-194)* _____

   _____

5. Describe three nursing measures to promote comfort in a woman who has an episiotomy or perineal laceration. *(177-178)*

   a. _____

   b. _____

   c. _____

6. Two separate incisions are done in cesarean delivery. What are they? Which of the two is more important and why? *(181)*

   _____

   _____

7. What nursing observations are appropriate after cesarean birth in each of the following areas and why? *(184)*

   a. Vital signs and other types of monitoring _____

   _____

   b. IV infusion _____

   _____

   c. Uterine fundus _____

   _____

   d. Dressing _____

   _____

   e. Lochia _____

   _____

Student Name _____

    f.   Indwelling catheter _____

    _____

8. Compare *hypertonic* labor to *hypotonic* labor for the following characteristics. Note which one is most common. *(184, 186-187)*

Characteristic	Hypertonic Labor	Hypotonic Labor
Contractions		
Time of occurrence during labor		
Medical management		
Nursing care		

9. Describe how each of the following factors can contribute to abnormal labor and list nursing measures appropriate for each.

    a.   Ineffective pushing efforts *(187)* _____

    _____

    _____

    _____

b. Occiput posterior fetal position *(187, 189-190)* _____

_____

_____

_____

10. State four ways that excessive psychological stress can contribute to a difficult labor. *(191)*

    a. _____

    b. _____

    c. _____

    d. _____

11. Describe possible adverse effects of prolonged labor on either the mother or the fetus. *(191)*

    a. _____

    b. _____

    c. _____

    d. _____

    e. _____

12. Describe possible adverse effects of precipitous labor on the mother and fetus. *(192)*

    a. _____

    b. _____

    c. _____

13. What is the difference between PROM and PPROM? *(192)*

    _____

    _____

    _____

    _____

14. What is the role of each of the following measures in the care of the woman with threatened or actual preterm labor? *(192, 194)*

    a. Transvaginal ultrasound _____

    _____

    b. Activity restrictions _____

    _____

    c. Fetal fibronectin _____

    _____

Student Name_____

15. Describe five or more symptoms of preterm labor that should be taught to every pregnant woman. List additional symptoms that you or a friend experienced if preterm labor occurred. *(193)*

_____

_____

_____

_____

_____

16. Describe nursing care of the fetus or neonate related to these problems of prolonged pregnancy. *(194)*

a. Placental blood supply _____

_____

b. Passage of meconium in utero _____

_____

c. Consumption of glucose reserves prior to birth _____

_____

17. Describe four situations in which the nurse must be especially watchful for a prolapsed umbilical cord. *(194-195)*

a. _____

b. _____

c. _____

d. _____

18. Describe three variations of uterine rupture. *(195)*

a. _____

_____

b. _____

_____

c. _____

_____

THINKING CRITICALLY

1. In addition to assessing the progress of labor, what other nursing assessments are important for the woman who has a precipitous labor? How can positioning the woman on her side improve the fetal oxygen supply?

CASE STUDIES

1. Cara Miller is a 24-year-old gravida 2, para 1, who is in early labor with her first baby. Her cervix is 3 cm dilated and 75% effaced; fetal station is 0. Contractions are every 4 minutes, 30–35 seconds in duration, and of moderate intensity. The nurse-midwife performs an amniotomy. A small amount of light-green fluid drains on the underpad.
    a. Use your birth facility's standard form as a worksheet to chart this information about Cara's labor. If the facility charts with a computer, write in the information that would be documented on computer.
    b. Is there significance to the color of the amniotic fluid? If so, what is the significance?
    c. What nursing interventions are appropriate specific to the situation above? Would other care providers in your facility be notified of these findings?
    d. Describe observations that would suggest that the amniotomy caused complications of any kind.

2. Baby boy Briggs was born in a forceps-assisted birth. What observations should the nurse make in each area listed below? What observations would be significant in terms of complications?
    a. Skin
    b. Shape of head
    c. Appearance when crying

3. Write a simple explanation to parents about the appearance of the infant's head if the birth was assisted with a vacuum extractor.

APPLYING KNOWLEDGE

1. Observe newborns who were in abnormal presentations or positions before birth. Identify characteristics caused by the abnormal presentation or position. Was the method of delivery vaginal (spontaneous or assisted by vacuum extractor or forceps) or cesarean? If cesarean birth, was it scheduled?

2. What nursing interventions do nurses in your clinical setting use when a mother is having complicated labor? How did you contribute to a mother's physical or psychological comfort during labor? What was the reason for the woman's abnormal labor?

3. What drugs to stop preterm labor are prescribed in your clinical setting? Read the policies and procedures related to administration of the drugs. If possible, assist in the care of a woman who is receiving the drugs. What concerns do the woman and her family express? If preterm labor contractions stop, does the woman remain in the hospital or is she discharged?

4. Make a list of activities appropriate for a woman on activity restriction for preterm labor, both in the hospital and at home.

5. How does your clinical facility determine if a woman's membranes have ruptured? Would additional tests would be done if she is at 30 weeks of gestation? Why?

6. Observe a woman who has a cesarean birth after labor, focusing on her feelings about the surgical birth. Compare your observations with those of classmates who have cared for other women who had scheduled cesarean births.

Student Name_____

REVIEW QUESTIONS

1. After amniotomy, which of the following observations should be reported immediately? *(174, 194)*
   1. Clear fluid draining on the underpad
   2. Maternal temperature of 37.2° C (99.0° F)
   3. Fetal heart rate of 95 bpm
   4. Moderate contractions every 3 minutes

2. Which is the most appropriate nursing care for the woman having hypertonic labor? *(184, 186)*
   1. Encourage walking in the hallway to improve contractions and enhance labor.
   2. Promote rest and provide general comfort measures.
   3. Reassure her that this problem will go away when active labor begins.
   4. Omit oral fluids and increase the rate of intravenous fluid.

3. A woman, gravida 4, para 3, has been 5 cm dilated for 2 hours. Her contractions are every 7 minutes, 30 seconds duration, and mild. The FHR is 135–145/minute. She is relatively comfortable. This woman is most likely experiencing: *(186)*
   1. hypotonic labor dysfunction.
   2. hypertonic labor dysfunction.
   3. occiput posterior fetal position.
   4. fetal shoulder dystocia.

4. The most desirable maternal position if prolapse of the umbilical cord occurs is: *(194-195)*
   1. side-lying.
   2. semi-Fowler's.
   3. Trendelenburg.
   4. knee-chest.

5. After a vaginal birth complicated by shoulder dystocia, the nurse should particularly assess the newborn for: *(187)*
   1. molding of the head.
   2. flexed positioning.
   3. clavicle deformity.
   4. abnormal temperature.

6. A woman has ruptured membranes at 31 weeks gestation. Which nursing observation should be promptly reported? *(192)*
   1. FHR: accelerations present; average rate of 145 bpm
   2. Small quantity of clear, nonirritating vaginal discharge
   3. Spontaneous fetal movement with uterine palpation
   4. Maternal vital signs: T 38.2° C (100.7° F), P 102, R 20

7. Which is the most typical labor characteristic when the fetus is in an occiput posterior position? *(187, 189)*
   1. Labor length under 3 hours
   2. Persistent back discomfort
   3. Rapid fetal descent
   4. Mild contraction strength

8. A woman who is at 32 weeks gestation telephones the nurse in a labor unit and says that her baby seems to be "pushing down" much of the time and that she has a constant backache. Choose the most appropriate nursing response. *(192-194)*
   1. Ask her to have someone bring her to the labor unit for further assessment.
   2. Reassure her that pressure and backache are common during late pregnancy.
   3. Tell her she should rest with her feet elevated several times each day.
   4. Encourage her to promote bladder emptying by increasing her fluid intake.

9. External version is most likely to be done in which of these situations? *(176-177)*
   1. Early labor with frank breech presentation
   2. Breech presentation with placenta previa
   3. Twins in cephalic and breech presentations
   4. Breech presentation at 38 weeks gestation

10. The first nursing action if a visibly prolapsed umbilical cord occurs is to: *(194-195)*
    1. call the physician or nurse-midwife.
    2. palpate the cord for a pulse.
    3. apply the internal fetal monitor.
    4. relieve pressure on the cord.

11. What is the priority nursing action following amniotomy? *(173-174)*
    1. Turn the woman to her side.
    2. Check the fetal heart rate.
    3. Assess the color of the fluid.
    4. Change the underpad.

12. The nursing intervention most likely to make the woman with a perineal laceration more comfortable during the first 2 hours after birth is: *(177-178)*
    1. warm-water soaks.
    2. a small dressing.
    3. an ice pack.
    4. antibacterial ointment.

13. Parents of a newborn delivered with low forceps ask about small bruises on each side of the baby's head. The nurse should tell the parents that the bruises: *(178-180)*
    1. will be reported to the physician.
    2. usually disappear in a few days.
    3. may indicate brain damage.
    4. occur in all vertex births.

14. Of the following options for cesarean birth, the most important nursing care during the postanesthesia recovery is to: *(184)*
    1. provide analgesia.
    2. assess the fundus.
    3. position for comfort.
    4. encourage urination.

Student Name_____

15. When caring for a woman following a vehicle accident at 36 weeks of pregnancy, the priority fetal assessment should be for: *(195-196)*
    1. undetected trauma.
    2. poor oxygenation.
    3. intrauterine infection.
    4. precipitous birth.

16. The nurse must particularly observe for signs and symptoms of uterine rupture if the laboring woman just admitted at 8 cm has: *(195-196)*
    1. a hypotonic labor pattern.
    2. a prior cesarean birth.
    3. prematurely ruptured membranes.
    4. estimated fetal weight of 3500 g.

17. An infant's amniotic fluid was meconium-stained. During the admission assessment, the nurse notes that the infant is crying vigorously. Her skin is peeling and she has a long, thin appearance. These facts suggest that this infant is probably: *(194)*
    1. preterm.
    2. postterm.
    3. in respiratory distress.
    4. large for her gestational age.

18. A woman has prostaglandin vaginal insert placed the day before she is scheduled for induction of labor at 40 weeks. Which is the most appropriate teaching immediately after the procedure? *(175)*
    1. We will check your baby's heart rate after you walk for 30 minutes.
    2. Expect vigorous and frequent contractions in about 30 minutes.
    3. Call your nurse if you notice fluid leaking from your vagina.
    4. Stay in bed on your left side until oxytocin infusion is started.

19. An infant is born by elective (planned) cesarean birth because of a breech presentation. The infant weighs 3206 g (7 pounds, 1 ounce). The nursery nurse should particularly observe this infant for: *(180)*
    1. low blood sugar.
    2. respiratory difficulty.
    3. birth injury.
    4. generalized infection.

Student Name _____

CHAPTER 9

The Family After Birth

Answer Key: Textbook page references are provided as a guide for answering these questions. A complete answer key was provided for your instructor.

LEARNING ACTIVITIES

1. Describe the following expected assessments for the uterine fundus immediately after birth. *(200-202)*

   a. Location _____

   b. Consistency _____

2. Describe the initial nursing action if the fundus is boggy (soft) and bleeding is excessive during the post-partum period. How does this action control uterine bleeding? *(202)*

   _____

   _____

3. List two drugs that may be ordered to correct uterine atony and the acceptable routes of administration. Does your facility use other drugs for more severe bleeding? *(202)*

   a. _____

   b. _____

4. List and describe the three stages of lochia, including approximate duration of each. *(201-202)*

   a. _____

   _____

   b. _____

   _____

   c. _____

   _____

5. When should perineal care be done? *(204)*

   a. _____

   b. _____

6. What should the nurse teach a postpartum woman about doing perineal care and about applying and removing her perineal pad? Why is it important to do these procedures in this way? *(204)*

   _____

   _____

7. a. The new mother can expect her menstrual periods to resume in _____ weeks if she is not breastfeeding. *(204)*

   b. In the breastfeeding mother, return of ovulation and menstruation are _____. *(204)*

8. Average blood loss at birth is about _____ for vaginal birth and _____ for cesarean birth. *(206)*

9. Describe two nursing actions that may make a woman who is chilled and shaking after birth more comfortable. *(206)*

   a. _____

   b. _____

10. Describe two possible signs of a full bladder in the immediate postpartum period. *(201, 203)*

    a. Height of uterus _____

    b. Location of uterus _____

11. Describe five nursing actions to help a new mother to empty her bladder after birth. *(207)*

    a. _____

    b. _____

    c. _____

    d. _____

    e. _____

12. List three nursing measures to prevent or correct constipation after birth. *(207)*

    a. _____

    b. _____

    c. _____

13. Describe each of the following factors about postbirth use of $Rh_o(D)$ immune globulin (RhoGAM). *(208)*

    a. Mother's Rh factor _____

    b. Infant's Rh factor _____

    c. Recommended time of administration after birth _____

    d. Site and route of administration _____

Student Name_____

14. Explain each of the following factors about postpartum rubella immunization. *(208)*

    a. Why it is given to the nonimmune woman at this time? _____

    _____

    b. Precautions _____

    _____

    c. Safety during breastfeeding _____

    _____

15. What assessments should the nurse make in each of these areas when caring for the woman who has had a cesarean birth? *(208-210)*

    a. Uterine fundus _____

    _____

    b. Lochia _____

    _____

    c. Dressing _____

    _____

    d. Urinary output _____

    _____

16. Name and describe Rubin's three postpartum psychological phases. *(211)*

    a. _____

    _____

    b. _____

    _____

    c. _____

    _____

17. What are the appropriate nursing interventions for postpartum blues? *(211)*

    _____

    _____

18. Describe nursing interventions that may be appropriate for grieving families in the maternity setting. If you wish, describe interventions that you or a family member or friend have experienced with grief, including grief other than infant loss. *(212-213)*

_____

_____

_____

_____

_____

19. Describe newborn behaviors during each phase of transition and the approximate duration of each stage. *(215)*

    a. First phase _____

_____

    b. Second phase _____

_____

    c. Third phase _____

_____

20. Why is prevention of neonatal hypothermia particularly important? *(215)*

_____

_____

21. How many arteries are in the newborn's umbilical cord? _____ How many veins? _____ What word can be used to help remember these numbers? _____ *(218)*

22. a. What is the minimum normal blood glucose on screening tests for a newborn (include units of measure)? _____ *(218-219)*

    b. List signs of hypoglycemia in a newborn. *(218-219)* _____

_____

_____

_____

23. List seven common laboratory screening tests for newborns. Identify the one that is mandatory in all states. List additional newborn screening tests that are offered in your clinical facility and whether they are mandatory or optional. *(219-220)*

    a. _____

    b. _____

Student Name_____

c. _____

d. _____

e. _____

f. _____

g. _____

Other: _____

24. List three types of parent-infant contact that enhance attachment. Which of these is most important? *(220)*

a. _____

b. _____

c. _____

25. a. Describe colostrum. *(222-224)* _____

_____

b. Explain the neonatal benefits of colostrum. *(222-224)* _____

_____

26. Describe methods to prevent and relieve breast engorgement. *(228-229)*

_____

_____

_____

27. Describe the following nutritional needs of the breastfeeding mother. *(230)*

a. Calories _____

b. Foods _____

c. Fluids _____

d. Supplements _____

28. What should the nurse teach the breastfeeding mother in each of the following areas? *(230)*

a. Foods that the infant may not tolerate _____

_____

b. Medications _____

_____

29. List four types of infant formula. Give an example of the three main types. *(231)*

    a. _____

    b. _____

    c. _____

    d. _____

30. Describe the three common forms for infant formulas. *(231)*

    _____

    _____

    _____

31. Describe teaching in each of the following areas for bottle-feeding parents. *(231-232, Skill 9-7)*

    a. Propping the bottle _____

    b. Size of nipple holes _____

    c. Warming and microwaving _____

    d. Burping _____

    e. Positioning baby after feeding _____

    f. Leftover formula _____

32. Describe appropriate nursing teaching in the following areas for postpartum discharge. *(233)*

    a. Hygiene _____

    _____

    b. Sexual intercourse _____

    _____

    c. Diet _____

    _____

33. List nine danger signals that a postpartum woman should promptly report to her physician or nurse midwife. *(233)*

    a. _____

    b. _____

Student Name _____

    c. _____

    d. _____

    e. _____

    f. _____

    g. _____

    h. _____

    i. _____

34. Describe the following factors about automobile safety. *(233-234)*

    a. Ideal position for infant _____

    b. When a forward-facing seat can be used _____

    c. Securing infant in seat and seat to vehicle _____

    d. Air bag safety _____

THINKING CRITICALLY

1. After a cesarean birth, what are some nursing interventions to help a mother manage pain while remaining alert enough to nurse her baby? Why is this mother likely to need additional nutrition teaching? What if her cesarean was done for placenta previa complicated by hemorrhage?

CASE STUDY

1. a. Cynthia Chung, 26 years old, expects her first baby in about 12 weeks. She says that she is having a difficult time deciding whether to breastfeed or bottle feed the baby. What information should you provide Cynthia to help her make this decision? What information would be available to use at your clinical facility?

    b. Cynthia decides to breastfeed her baby. On the fifth day after birth, she phones the unit to say that she has breast engorgement and her nipples are sore. Her left nipple has a small crack. What can the nurse teach Cynthia to help her cope with these problems?

    c. What should the nurse teach Cynthia about care of the baby's umbilical stump? What signs of problems should she report?

APPLYING KNOWLEDGE

1. What analgesics do postpartum women in your hospital receive for pain? Do nurses use any nonpharmacologic techniques to make the women more comfortable?

2. Observe families during the postpartum period. What interactions do you see among mother, father, and newborn? Identify practices in your clinical setting that enhance or inhibit parent-infant attachment.

3. Assist the staff nurse to help new mothers learn to breastfeed. If you have successfully breastfed a baby yourself, share appropriate helpful hints with new mothers and classmates.

4. Identify the protocol in your clinical facility for checking newborn glucose levels.
    a. Newborns who are routinely screened?
    b. Routine times for screening?
    c. Interventions for abnormal newborn glucose levels?

5. Role-play with a classmate how to discuss the choice of breastfeeding or formula feeding with a pregnant woman.

REVIEW QUESTIONS

1. Which of the following postpartum patient assessments requires immediate nursing intervention? *(201-202)*
    1. Excretion of large amounts of urine on first postpartum day
    2. Soft uterine fundus, to right of the midline, 2 hours after birth
    3. Nipples intact but reddened on the first postpartum day
    4. Perineal area edematous with minor tenderness and slight bruising

2. The most serious potential problem if a woman's bladder is distended in the early postpartum period is: *(202, 207)*
    1. infection.
    2. discomfort.
    3. vomiting.
    4. hemorrhage.

3. Which of these women is most likely to have afterpains? *(201)*
    1. gravida 1, para 1, 6.5 lb (2951 g) infant
    2. gravida 3, para 1, 7 lb (3178 g) infant
    3. gravida 1, para 1, twins weighing 3.5 lb (1589 g) and 4.5 lb (2043 g)
    4. gravida 4, para 4, 9.5 lb (4313 g) infant

4. Two hours after a woman's uncomplicated vaginal birth requiring no anesthesia, the nurse notes that her uterus is firm, two fingerwidths above her umbilicus, and deviated slightly to her right side. The most appropriate nursing action at this time is to: *(207)*
    1. check her blood pressure and pulse.
    2. massage her uterus continuously.
    3. insert an indwelling catheter.
    4. help her walk to the bathroom to urinate.

Student Name_____

5. Choose the situation that describes appropriate administration of Rh$_o$(D) immune globulin (RhoGAM). *(208)*
   1. Rh-negative infant, Rh-negative mother, given IV to the infant within 12 hours of birth
   2. Rh-positive infant, Rh-negative mother, given IV to the mother within 1 week of birth
   3. Rh-positive infant, Rh-negative mother, given IM to the mother within 72 hours of birth
   4. Rh-negative infant, Rh-positive mother, given IM to the mother within 72 hours of birth

6. When teaching parents about PKU testing, the nurse should teach them that: *(219)*
   1. a negative test indicates that their baby will not have brain damage.
   2. follow-up testing should be done during one of the early clinic visits.
   3. the test must be done before the infant nurses or has any formula.
   4. a special diet started with solid foods will prevent disability.

7. The nurse gives a postpartum woman a rubella immunization. Which is the most important patient teaching related to this immunization? *(208)*
   1. Neomycin can be used for rash or elevated temperature.
   2. Use a reliable birth control method for 3 months.
   3. Immunization now gives the baby immunity through breast milk.
   4. Increased urination is a common side effect of the immunization.

8. What should the mother be taught about perineal cleansing? *(204)*
   1. Do perineal cleansing only after bowel movements.
   2. Cleanse from back to front with soft wipes.
   3. Direct the flow of fluid from the front to the back.
   4. Avoid disposable wipes on the perineal area.

9. Colostrum's greatest benefit to the infant is prevention of: *(222)*
   1. constipation.
   2. weight loss.
   3. hemorrhage.
   4. infection.

10. The let-down reflex is stimulated by: *(223, Table 9-2, 226-227)*
    1. massage of the uterus.
    2. suckling of the baby.
    3. increased fluid intake.
    4. breast engorgement.

11. What should the nursing mother be taught about breast care? *(205-206)*
    1. Clean the breasts with plain water when washing.
    2. Give one formula feeding daily to limit engorgement.
    3. Do not wear a bra the first few days after birth.
    4. Begin with the same breast at each feeding.

12. Parents should be taught that the safest position for their term newborn in the crib is: *(217)*
    1. with the head elevated.
    2. side-lying with head down.
    3. on either the back or side.
    4. prone with head elevated.

13. At her 2-week postpartum checkup, the woman's uterus should be: *(200-201)*
    1. two fingerwidths above the umbilicus.
    2. two fingerwidths below the umbilicus.
    3. just above the symphysis pubis.
    4. no longer palpable through the abdomen.

14. Diuresis in the early postpartum period indicates: *(206)*
    1. urinary tract infection.
    2. retention of body fluids.
    3. excretion of excess fluid.
    4. edema near the urinary meatus.

15. The earliest time when sexual intercourse can usually be resumed after birth is: *(233)*
    1. at 2 weeks postpartum.
    2. when the episiotomy heals.
    3. when lochia alba is present.
    4. after the 6-week check.

16. The most appropriate way to identify mother and infant when reuniting them is to: *(216)*
    1. check the identification band numbers of each.
    2. ask the mother to clearly state her name.
    3. examine the mother's fingerprint and infant's footprints.
    4. verify that the names on the crib card and band are identical.

17. Which is the best nursing measure to increase the woman's perineal comfort during the first hour after vaginal birth with a midline episiotomy? *(204)*
    1. Help her take a warm sitz bath.
    2. Give her an oral analgesic drug.
    3. Apply topical anesthetic ointment.
    4. Place an ice pack on the area.

18. A mother phones the postpartum unit 4 days after birth. She says her baby cannot suck well on her nipples because her breasts are full and engorged. What should the nurse recommend? *(205-206, 227)*
    1. Apply ice packs just before allowing the infant to nurse.
    2. Feed formula for the next two feedings to reduce pain and congestion.
    3. Massage the breasts and express a small amount of milk before nursing.
    4. Reduce daily liquid intake to 1 quart for a few days.

19. The nurse notes that a new mother has several bottles of partly consumed formula on her overbed table. Choose the most appropriate nursing action. *(230-232, Skill 9-7)*
    1. Recommend that she prepare bottles that contain only what the baby is likely to drink.
    2. Inform her that the bottles cannot be used because they have not been refrigerated.
    3. Tell her she may combine the leftover formula for the baby's next feeding.
    4. Check the room for other partially used bottles, then throw all of them in the trash.

20. Which lochia characteristic should the nurse teach the woman to report? *(202)*
    1. Change from red to pink-brown to white
    2. Cessation of flow by 4 weeks postpartum
    3. Return of red flow at 12 days postpartum
    4. Presence of a menstrual-like odor

CROSSWORD PUZZLE

Student Name_____

Across

3. Heat loss caused when infant is placed on cool surface for assessment *(215)*
6. Acronym used for assessment of episiotomy or other incision *(203-204)*
7. Vaginal drainage after birth that has three stages *(201-202)*
9. Lochia that has a pink color *(201)*
12. Abbreviation for intrauterine growth restriction *(217)*
13. Bloody postpartum lochia *(201)*
14. Drug used to reverse respiratory depression caused by epidural narcotics *(210)*
15. Human milk having a bluish color *(224)*
17. Heat loss caused by locating infant's crib near a cold wall *(215)*
18. Breast milk enhancers used by some cultures *(224)*
22. Direction the infant should face in his or her car seat *(233-234)*
23. Mood instability *(211)*
26. Return of uterus to its normal state after birth *(200)*
27. Top of the uterus that contracts to control bleeding after birth *(200)*
28. Milk secreted after colostrum *(223-224)*
30. Strong emotional tie that develops soon after birth *(220)*
31. Separation of the longitudinal abdominal muscles (rectus muscles) *(207)*
32. Breast milk with higher fat content to satisfy infant's hunger *(223)*

Down

1. Father's intense interest in his new baby *(211)*
2. Anterior pituitary hormone that stimulates breast to produce milk *(223)*
4. First breast secretion; high in antibodies *(223-224)*
5. First 6 weeks after birth *(199)*
8. Intermittent uterine contractions after birth; similar to menstrual cramps *(201)*
9. Giving or taking nourishment at the breast *(226)*
10. Heat loss caused by air-conditioning vent blowing air on infant *(215)*
11. Good infant hold for breastfeeding woman who had cesarean birth *(224-225)*
16. Long-term affection tie between the infant and parent *(220)*
19. Lochia that is mostly mucus *(201)*
20. Posterior pituitary hormone that causes let-down reflex and uterine contractions *(223)*
21. Heat loss caused when parent bathes infant slowly *(215)*
24. Reflex that ejects milk from alveoli to the ductal system of nipple *(223)*
25. Watery, thirst-quenching breast milk *(223)*
29. Vaginal folds *(203)*
30. Brief feelings of joy and emotional letdown after birth *(211)*

CHAPTER 10

Nursing Care of Women with Complications Following Birth

Answer Key: Textbook page references are provided as a guide for answering these questions. A complete answer key was provided for your instructor.

LEARNING ACTIVITIES

1. Match the terms in the left column with their definitions on the right (a–m).

_____ "Baby blues" *(246)*	a. Infection of the uterine lining
_____ Bipolar disorder *(247)*	b. Infection of the breast
_____ Curettage *(241, 246)*	c. Lodging of a blood clot in a blood vessel of the lung
_____ Postpartum depression *(246-247)*	d. Calf pain when the foot is dorsiflexed
_____ Endometritis *(243)*	e. Inadequate amount of blood to maintain normal circulation
_____ Hematoma *(241)*	f. Mood disorder characterized by impairment of reality
_____ Homans' sign *(242)*	g. Mood disorder characterized by episodes of mania alternating with depression
_____ Hypovolemic shock *(236-237)*	h. Hyperactive, excitable, euphoric behavior
_____ Mania *(247)*	i. Delayed return of the uterus to its nonpregnant state
_____ Mastitis *(244-245, 246)*	j. Collection of blood within tissues
_____ Psychosis *(246)*	k. Scraping or vacuuming the inner surface of the uterus
_____ Pulmonary embolism *(242)*	l. Postpartum emotional state characterized by feelings of being let down, but generally satisfied with life
_____ Subinvolution *(245-246)*	m. Non-psychosis characterized by loss of enjoyment, lack of interest, feelings of inadequacy after birth

2. Postpartum hemorrhage is blood loss that exceeds _____ ml after vaginal birth or _____ ml after cesarean birth. *(236)*

3. Early postpartum hemorrhage occurs within _____ hours of birth; late postpartum hemorrhage occurs later than _____ hours after birth until _____ weeks after birth. *(236)*

4. Describe the following five changes that occur in hypovolemic shock and indicate the change or changes that usually occur early. *(236-237)*

    a. Heart rate _____

    _____

    b. Respiratory rate _____

    _____

    c. Blood pressure _____

    _____

    d. Skin and mucous membranes _____

    _____

    e. Mental state _____

    _____

5. Why does a poorly contracted uterus lead to hemorrhage? *(237, 239-240)*

    _____

    _____

6. What is the connection between the infant suckling at the breast and control of postpartum bleeding? *(240)*

    _____

    _____

7. Describe typical differences in bleeding and uterine fundus characteristics between hemorrhage caused by uterine atony and that caused by a birth canal laceration. *(240-241)*

    a. Bleeding

    Uterine atony _____

    _____

    Laceration _____

    _____

    b. Uterine fundus

    Uterine atony _____

    _____

    _____

Laceration _____

_____

_____

8. Describe the following typical manifestations of a birth canal hematoma. *(241)*

a. Visual appearance _____

_____

b. Character of pain or pressure _____

_____

_____

c. Signs of blood loss _____

_____

9. How does manual removal of the placenta differ from the usual method of separation? *(241)*

_____

_____

10. Distinguish between the characteristics of a superficial vein thrombosis (SVT) and a deep vein thrombosis (DVT). *(241-243)*

a. Superficial vein thrombosis _____

_____

b. Deep vein thrombosis _____

_____

11. The greatest risk of deep vein thrombosis is that it may result in _____
_____. *(241-243)*

12. Postpartum infection is generally characterized by a temperature of _____ after the first _____
hours after birth, occurring on at least _____ days during the first _____ days after birth. *(243)*

13. List the localized signs and symptoms of an infection such as a wound infection. *(243, Table 10-3)*

_____

_____

14. Why are postpartum infections in the reproductive tract likely to spread? *(243-244)*

_____

_____

15. Why may the white blood cell (leukocyte) count be unreliable as the only assessment to diagnose infection after birth? *(244)*

    _____

16. What nutritional information is important when teaching the woman who has—or is at an increased risk of having—a postpartum infection? Would this teaching be appropriate for other people with an infection? *(244)*

    _____

    _____

17. Distinguish between *cystitis* and *pyelonephritis* in terms of the following characteristics. Which is the most serious? *(243, Table 10-3)*

    a. Fever _____

    _____

    b. Discomfort _____

    _____

    c. Other characteristics _____

    _____

18. Describe the following nursing measures to promote recovery from urinary tract infection and prevent future ones. *(243)*

    a. Fluid intake _____

    _____

    b. Beneficial foods _____

    _____

19. Which two factors increase the likelihood that mastitis will develop? *(243, 244-245)*

    a. _____

    b. _____

20. What is the role of heat application in the care of a woman with mastitis? *(244-245)*

    a. _____

    b. _____

    c. _____

21. Describe three characteristics of subinvolution of the uterus. *(245)*

    a. _____

    _____

Student Name _____

    b. _____

         _____

    c. _____

         _____

22. Describe the basic difference between postpartum "blues" and postpartum depression. *(246-247)*

    a. Postpartum "blues" _____

         _____

         _____

    b. Postpartum depression _____

         _____

         _____

THINKING CRITICALLY

1. How can the nurse's teaching about breastfeeding reduce the likelihood that a woman will develop mastitis? Give examples of what you might teach the mother of a term newborn.

2. A woman is having her 6-week examination after a normal vaginal birth at the office where you work. She has a "flat" appearance to her face and seems uninterested in what you say to her, although she cooperates with each request related to her examination and cares for her baby when he cries. What possibilities for her behavior should you consider? How should you respond to her?

CASE STUDY

1. Carmen Esparza is transferred to the mother-baby unit after a cesarean delivery 2 hours ago following a long labor. Her healthy daughter weighs 4540 g (10 pounds). Carmen's blood loss during surgery was 1200 ml. Her vital signs on admission to the unit are: T 99° F, P 86, R 20, BP 118/80. Her fundus is firm, midline, and lochia is scant in amount. The dressing over her incision is clean and dry. The indwelling catheter bag contained 550 ml of light-yellow urine when it was emptied before transfer from the recovery room. Carmen is awake and says she is "really tired." She received epidural morphine (Duramorph) prior to leaving the operating room and rates her pain as 0 on a pain scale. (Use information from Chapters 7, 9, and 10 to answer the questions in this exercise.)
    a. Identify the priority nursing diagnosis for Carmen during her recovery period. What interventions are appropriate for this nursing diagnosis? What other important nursing diagnosis should be considered? Why?
    b. Carmen's vital signs are: T 98.6° F, P 96, R 20, BP 110/90 1 hour later. Lochia is moderate, with some small clots. Her catheter bag contains a very small amount of urine. She is slightly restless, but says she has no pain. How should you interpret these assessments? Do you need any other information? What action should you take?
    c. Are other complications more likely to develop later in the postpartum period? What do you think they would be?

APPLYING KNOWLEDGE

1. Look at the vital sign charts (including pulse oximetry if available) of several postpartum women. What is the pattern of their temperature and pulse rates after birth? Do you see any differences in these patterns among women who had a vaginal birth and those who had a cesarean birth? Can you see any effects of labor medication on vital signs?

2. Study the routine postpartum teaching given to all women before discharge. For each sign or symptom that a woman should report, identify the complications related to that sign or symptom.

3. Determine if your clinical facility provides written postpartum self-care instructions in languages other than English. If not, what provisions does the staff make for patients who do not speak English?

4. Ask if your clinical facility provides new mothers with information about postpartum depression. If provided, where is it documented? Watch an RN provide this information if possible.

REVIEW QUESTIONS

1. A woman had a forceps-assisted birth 2 hours ago. Baseline vital signs were T 37.1° C (98.8° F), P 78, R 20, BP 118/70. Which of the following assessments suggests possible development of hypovolemic shock in this woman? *(236-237)*
   1. Firm fundus, slightly right of midline
   2. Pulse 100, respirations 24
   3. Respirations 22, blood pressure 114/76
   4. Light lochia rubra with small clots

2. A woman had a 16-hour labor that ended with the cesarean birth of a 4313 g (9.5 lb) infant. Her membranes were ruptured for 24 hours and oxytocin augmentation of labor was attempted before the cesarean birth. She has an IV infusion of Ringers' lactate and an indwelling catheter. For which complication should the nurse be most observant during the immediate recovery-room period? *(237, 239-241)*
   1. Uterine atony
   2. Endometritis
   3. Uterine subinvolution
   4. Urinary tract infection

3. If the nurse finds that a new mother's uterus is soft, the appropriate initial action is to: *(240)*
   1. insert an indwelling catheter.
   2. massage the uterus until it is firm.
   3. check the woman's vital signs.
   4. increase the rate of the IV fluid.

4. One hour after vaginal birth, the nurse notes that a woman has a flat purple area, about 2 cm by 3 cm, on her perineum. Which is the most appropriate nursing action at this time? *(241, Table 10-1)*
   1. Assist her to take a warm sitz bath.
   2. Apply pressure with a tightly applied pad.
   3. Reapply a chemical cold pack on the area.
   4. Notify the physician of the observation.

5. When teaching a woman following vaginal birth 24 hours ago, the nurse should tell her to report: *(241, 245)*
   1. pink vaginal drainage followed by red drainage.
   2. menstrual-like odor of vaginal discharge.
   3. uterine cramping when the infant nurses.
   4. excretion of large quantities of dilute urine.

Student Name_____

6. Choose the most appropriate intervention to prevent deep vein thrombosis in a woman who is one day post-cesarean birth. *(242-243)*
   1. Encourage her to walk several times each day.
   2. Provide her with increased fluids that she enjoys.
   3. Take her temperature to identify an elevation.
   4. Instruct her to stay in bed most of the day.

7. Choose the finding that suggests infection after birth. *(243-244)*
   1. Poorly relieved perineal pain 4 hours postpartum
   2. Oral temperature of 37.7° C (100° F) 18 hours postpartum
   3. White blood cell count of 21,000/dl at 1 day postpartum
   4. Persistent and severe cramping 3 days postpartum

8. The best position for the woman who has postpartum endometritis is: *(243-244, Table 10-3)*
   1. semisitting.
   2. side-lying.
   3. supine.
   4. prone.

9. Which nursing assessment suggests that a postpartum woman has cystitis? *(243, Table 10-3)*
   1. Burning with every urination
   2. High fever accompanied by chills
   3. Fever with nausea and vomiting
   4. Voiding large amounts of urine

10. Which nurse's teaching is appropriate for the new mother who has cystitis? *(243, Table 10-3)*
    1. Eat several servings of whole grains and meats each day.
    2. Remain in bed except for going to the bathroom.
    3. Drink about 3 liters of noncaffeinated beverages daily.
    4. Take a stool softener to reduce added pain of constipation.

11. A woman is 8 hours postpartum after a spontaneous vaginal birth. Her admission hemoglobin was 9.5 g/dl, and her estimated blood loss during the birth was 1000 ml. She asks the nurse if she can walk to the bathroom. The best nursing response is to: *(237)*
    1. remind her that she should catch her urine in a "hat" to be measured.
    2. have her sit briefly on the side of the bed before helping her to the bathroom.
    3. encourage her to urinate every 2 hours to decrease the risk of excess bleeding.
    4. tell her to return to bed promptly after she finishes using the bathroom.

12. Which nursing assessment suggests infection of an episiotomy? *(243, Table 10-3)*
    1. Temperature of 37.8° C (100° F) 12 hours after birth
    2. Purplish discoloration of the perineum and labia
    3. Edema of the labia minora, labia majora, and perineum
    4. Redness of the perineum with separation of the suture line

13. A woman has postpartum uterine atony with hemorrhage. After bleeding is controlled, the physician orders an indwelling catheter mainly because it: *(237)*
    1. allows better estimation of the woman's blood volume.
    2. identifies bloody urine that suggests bladder trauma.
    3. limits the need for the woman to ambulate to the bathroom.
    4. applies constant pressure against the bleeding uterus.

14. A woman who is 3 days postpartum comes to the emergency clinic because she is having pain and burning discomfort when she urinates. She denies that she has had any fever and states that her lochia is "light pink." The nurse should expect an initial order for: *(243-244)*
    1. bladder analgesics.
    2. intravenous antibiotics.
    3. culture of vaginal discharge.
    4. clean-catch urine specimen.

15. A woman is 5 days postpartum and breastfeeding. She telephones the nurse at the clinic and says that her breasts feel very heavy and one of them is tender. She says the infant nurses "fair." The nurse should tell the woman that: *(244-246)*
    1. her symptoms should go away when the infant begins nursing better.
    2. breastfeeding should be stopped until the pain goes away.
    3. a cold pack between feedings should reduce the pain.
    4. she should come to the clinic for evaluation of her symptoms.

16. Methylergonovine (Methergine) should be avoided if the woman has: *(240)*
    1. uterine atony.
    2. retained placenta.
    3. hypertension.
    4. endometritis.

17. Select the woman who is at greatest risk for bleeding from a vaginal wall laceration. *(240-241)*
    1. Vaginal birth assisted with vacuum extractor
    2. First infant who weighs 3632 g (8 lb)
    3. History of uterine atony with previous birth
    4. Oxytocin (Pitocin) used to induce labor

18. Choose the foods that are highest in iron. *(244)*
    1. Citrus fruits, apricots, tomatoes
    2. Sweet and white potatoes, corn, dried beans
    3. Enriched bread, dark green leafy vegetables
    4. Milk, cheeses, legumes

19. A woman comes to the clinic for her 6-week postpartum check after having her first baby. She says to the nurse, "I don't know what's wrong with me. I'm exhausted all the time and yet I can't seem to sleep when I have the chance." The nurse should: *(246)*
    1. reassure her that the demands of being a mother can seem overwhelming, especially with the first baby.
    2. ask her if her partner, family members, or friends can help her with care of the baby and her home so she can rest.
    3. explain that women lose more blood at birth than they expect, and a slight anemia often leads to these symptoms.
    4. find a quiet place to talk with her about her feelings related to her new role as a mother.

20. Postpartum bipolar disorder is characterized by: *(247)*
    1. periods of let-down feelings but with general enjoyment of life.
    2. impaired reality characterized by euphoria alternating with depression.
    3. alternate periods of overeating and lack of interest in food and drink.
    4. prolonged feelings of worthlessness or guilt.

CHAPTER 11

The Nurse's Role in Women's Health Care

Answer Key: Textbook page references are provided as a guide for answering these questions. A complete answer key was provided for your instructor.

LEARNING ACTIVITIES

1. Match the terms in the left column with their definitions on the right (a–r).

_____ Basal temperature *(259)*	a. Device inserted into vagina to support pelvic structures
_____ Climacteric *(272)*	b. Painful sexual intercourse
_____ Cystocele *(276)*	c. Presence of tissue resembling uterine lining outside the uterus
_____ Dyspareunia *(253)*	d. Release of semen into the male's bladder during sexual intercourse
_____ Endometriosis *(253)*	e. Stretching of the cervical mucus at ovulation
_____ Infertility *(268)*	f. Body temperature at rest, taken before any activity
_____ Libido *(273)*	g. Weak vaginal wall that cannot support the bladder properly
_____ Menopause *(272)*	h. Weak posterior vaginal wall that inhibits proper stool passage
_____ Myoma *(277)*	i. Inability to conceive when desired
_____ Osteoporosis *(273)*	j. Enlarged vein in the scrotum
_____ Pessary *(276)*	k. Unexpected loss of urine when laughing, coughing, or sneezing
_____ Rectocele *(276)*	l. Inability to control urge to urinate due to over-active bladder
_____ Retrograde ejaculation *(268)*	m. Cessation of menstruation
_____ Spinnbarkeit *(259-260)*	n. Benign tumors of the uterine muscle
_____ Stress incontinence *(276)*	o. Sexual desire
_____ Urge incontinence *(276)*	p. Period of time surrounding the cessation of menstruation
_____ Uterine prolapse *(276)*	q. Loss of bone mass leading to bone fragility
_____ Varicocele *(269)*	r. Weakened support ligaments for the vagina and uterus

2. a. The best time to perform breast self-examination is _____ or _____. *(250-251)*

b. Professional breast examination should be done _____ for all women over the age of _____. *(250-251)*

c. The American Cancer Society recommends that mammography be done for all women aged _____ at _____ intervals. *(250-251)*

3. List the preparation a woman should make before having a Pap test. *(251)*

a. _____

b. _____

4. a. The Pap test is recommended at _____ intervals for all women age _____ or older. *(251)*

b. Under what conditions can a Pap test be done less frequently? *(251)* _____

_____

5. Define each term that relates to menstrual disorders. *(252-253)*

a. Amenorrhea _____

b. Primary amenorrhea _____

c. Secondary amenorrhea _____

d. Metrorrhagia _____

e. Menorrhagia _____

f. Mittelschmerz _____

g. Dysmenorrhea _____

6. How can a low body weight contribute to amenorrhea? *(252)*

_____

_____

7. List common symptoms of premenstrual dysphoric disorder (PMDD). *(253)*

a. _____

b. _____

c. _____

d. _____

e. _____

f. _____

g. _____

h. _____

Student Name _____

    i.   _____

    j.   _____

    k.   _____

8.   a.   When do the symptoms of PMDD occur? *(253)* _____

         _____

    b.   How many of the typical symptoms are required to diagnose PMDD? *(253)* _____

         _____

    c.   Describe therapy that may be prescribed for PMDD. *(253)* _____

         _____

    d.   Explain nursing responsibilities related to PMDD. *(253)* _____

         _____

9.   List four factors that contribute to vaginal infection and why they increase this risk. *(253-254)*

    a.   _____

    b.   _____

    c.   _____

    d.   _____

10. Describe important teaching related to toxic shock syndrome in each area listed. *(254)*

    a.   Handwashing _____

         _____

         _____

    b.   Use of tampons _____

         _____

         _____

    c.   Use of cervical cap or diaphragm for contraception _____

         _____

         _____

11. a.   Describe signs and symptoms of candidiasis. *(255, Table 11-1)*

         _____

         _____

b. List common medications used to treat candidiasis. *(255, Table 11-1)*

_____

_____

12. a. What is the most prevalent viral sexually transmitted disease? *(257-258, Table 11-1)*

_____

b. What are the characteristics of this infection? *(257-258, Table 11-1)*

_____

_____

c. What complications may occur during birth or after birth for the infant? *(257-258, Table 11-1)*

_____

d. What malignant complication is associated with the infection and what precautions should the woman take related to this associated complication? *(257-258, Table 11-1)*

_____

_____

13. How can Chlamydia or gonorrhea infections result in infertility or an ectopic pregnancy? *(256-258, Table 11-1, 269)*

_____

_____

14. a. The STI (also called STD for sexually transmissible disease) that has three possible stages is _____. *(256, Table 11-1, 258)*

b. Describe the characteristics of each stage of this infection. *(256, Table 11-1, 258)*

Primary _____

_____

Secondary _____

_____

Tertiary _____

_____

c. What is the main drug used to treat it? Which alternate drug must be avoided during pregnancy? *(256, Table 11-1, 258)*

_____

_____

Student Name _____

15. Infections of _____ can reemerge later in outbreaks that are also infectious. *(257-258, Table 11-1)*

16. a. Most oral contraceptives contain _____ and _____, while some contain only _____. *(261)*

    b. How does this drug or combination of drugs prevent pregnancy? *(261)*_____

    _____

17. What is the significance of the ACHES acronym in relation to oral contraceptives? What does each letter stand for? *(261)*

    A _____

    C _____

    H _____

    E _____

    S _____

18. Depo-Provera provides _____ months of effective contraception. It is given by the _____ route within _____ days of the menstrual period. Why is this timing important? *(262)*

19. List the three most common side effects of Depo-Provera. *(262)*

    a. _____

    b. _____

    c. _____

20. What is the major difference among these intrauterine devices in terms of effectiveness? *(262)*

    a. Copper-containing (ParaGard) _____

    b. Levonorgestrel-releasing _____

21. List two times when the diaphragm must be refitted. *(263)*

    a. _____

    b. _____

22. Describe appropriate teaching about condom use in each area listed. *(265, Skill 11-3)*

    a. Lubrication _____

    _____

    b. Breakage or dislodgment during use _____

    _____

    c. Expiration date _____

    _____

    d. Removal _____

    _____

23. Describe three methods that can be used for natural family planning. *(259-260)*

    a. _____

    _____

    b. _____

    _____

    c. _____

    _____

24. Why must another form of contraception be used for about 1 month following vasectomy? *(267)*

    _____

    _____

25. Describe four types of emergency contraception, including administration. *(266)*

    a. Oral contraceptives or Preven kit _____

    _____

    b. Levonorgestrel _____

    _____

    c. Intrauterine device _____

    _____

    d. Mifepristone (RU 486) _____

    _____

26. a. Define *primary infertility.* *(268)* _____

    _____

    b. Define *secondary infertility.* *(268)* _____

    _____

27. Describe the psychological reactions a couple may have to infertility. *(268)*

    _____

    _____

    _____

    _____

    _____

Student Name _____

28. a. Describe how each male factor can compromise fertility. *(268-269)*

Abnormal sperm _____

_____

Abnormal erections _____

_____

Abnormal ejaculation _____

_____

Abnormal seminal fluid _____

_____

b. Describe how each female factor can compromise fertility. *(268-269)*

Disorders of ovulation _____

_____

Abnormalities of fallopian tubes _____

_____

Abnormalities of uterus, cervix, or ovaries _____

_____

Hormone abnormalities _____

_____

29. Describe similarities and differences among the following assisted reproductive techniques. *(270-271)*

a. In vitro fertilization (IVF) _____

_____

b. Gamete intrafallopian transfer (GIFT) _____

_____

c. Tubal embryo transfer (TET) _____

_____

d. Microsurgery _____

_____

30. Describe the following changes that may occur during the climacteric. *(272-273)*

a. Menstrual cycles _____

_____

b. Vasomotor instability _____

_____

c. Vaginal changes _____

_____

31. Describe changes in these structures that occur with loss of estrogen. *(272-273)*

a. Uterus and ovaries _____

_____

b. Vagina _____

_____

c. Pelvic musculature _____

_____

d. Bones _____

_____

32. a. Describe the advantages and risks of hormone replacement therapy (HRT). *(273)*

_____

_____

b. Explain conditions in which HRT is contraindicated. *(273)*

_____

_____

33. List six types of complementary therapy that may be used instead of, or as an alternative to, HRT and the purpose for each. *(273)*

a. _____

b. _____

c. _____

d. _____

e. _____

f. _____

34. Describe each variation of vaginal wall prolapse. *(276)*

a. Cystocele _____

_____

b. Rectocele _____

_____

Student Name_____

35. What treatments may be used to reduce symptomatic uterine myomas? *(277)*

    a. Medical treatment _____

    _____

    _____

    b. Surgical treatment _____

    _____

    _____

THINKING CRITICALLY

1. When in your orthopedic experience, note how many women are affected with hip fractures compared to the number of men affected. Does one ethnic group seem to be more affected than others? Do you notice signs of osteoporosis in these patients? What imaging techniques have been used to determine the location and severity of osteoporosis? Have you had a bone density scan?

APPLYING KNOWLEDGE

1. Interview nurses at a clinic about their experience caring for patients with STIs. Which diseases are most prevalent?

2. Under supervision, teach a woman to perform a breast self-examination (BSE).

3. Observe a mammogram. Are multiple imaging techniques used to better evaluate breast tissue?

REVIEW QUESTIONS

1. The nurse is teaching a woman, age 25, about BSE. The correct teaching is that BSE: *(250-251, Skill 11-1)*
    1. detects malignancy more often than professional examinations.
    2. allows her to delay the need for mammography until she is 50 years old.
    3. helps her learn the normal characteristics of her own breasts.
    4. is more accurate than a yearly mammogram.

2. Choose the correct teaching about BSE technique. *(250, Skill 11-1)*
    1. Use the palms of the hand to press the breast tissue firmly against the ribs.
    2. Palpate each breast systematically, using the pads of the fingers.
    3. Palpate the underarm area only if the breasts are very large or sagging.
    4. Squeeze the breast tissue between the thumb and index finger.

3. Choose the correct teaching for relief of symptoms associated with premenstrual dysphoric disorder. *(253)*
    1. Eat chocolate candies several times a day to reduce fluid retention and weight gain.
    2. Reduce fluid intake during the first half of the menstrual cycle.
    3. Plan the most stressful activities during the last half of the menstrual cycle.
    4. Exercise individually or with others several times each week.

4. When teaching about the use of tampons, the nurse should emphasize replacing them at least every 4 hours to prevent: *(254)*
   1. pelvic inflammatory disease.
   2. vasomotor symptoms.
   3. sexually transmitted infections.
   4. toxic shock syndrome.

5. A friend asks you what she can do because she is troubled by repeated "yeast" infections. As a nurse, your best advice to her is to: *(255, Table 11-1)*
   1. keep over-the-counter medications on hand so she can begin treatment immediately.
   2. see her medical caregiver if she has another infection to identify possible causes.
   3. increase her intake of fluids to include at least eight glasses of water each day.
   4. avoid sexual intercourse for 1 month to see if that reduces the infections.

6. The long-term risk of an infection with the human papillomavirus is for: *(258)*
   1. cervical cancer.
   2. ectopic pregnancy.
   3. endometriosis.
   4. nerve damage.

7. Other than abstinence, the best way to prevent sexually transmitted infection with the human immunodeficiency virus is: *(257-258)*
   1. douching within 30 minutes of sexual intercourse.
   2. avoiding intercourse during midcycle.
   3. use of a condom for all episodes of sexual intercourse.
   4. taking prophylactic antibiotics after unprotected intercourse.

8. Choose the most appropriate teaching for the woman who is prescribed multiphasic oral contraceptive pills. *(261)*
   1. The menstrual period begins when the fourth week of pills is completed.
   2. Cigarette smoking should be limited to no more than 10 per day.
   3. Limit intake of foods that are high in iron or calcium.
   4. Take the pills at the same time of day and in order.

9. Choose the woman who should not take oral contraceptives. *(261)*
   1. A woman who has multiple sexual partners.
   2. A 38-year-old woman who smokes a pack of cigarettes daily.
   3. A 19-year-old woman who is formula feeding her 2-month-old baby.
   4. A woman who is being discharged after a spontaneous abortion.

10. A woman has been taking oral contraceptives for 4 months. She is concerned because her periods are much lighter than before she started the pills. How should the nurse counsel this woman? *(261)*
    1. "You will probably have to discontinue the pill unless your periods become more like they were previously."
    2. "We can switch you to a barrier contraceptive; your periods should return to normal in just a few months."
    3. "Lighter periods are expected when you are on the pill but you should tell us if they stop entirely."
    4. "Stop taking the pills immediately. We want to do a pregnancy test before you resume them."

Student Name _____

11. Choose the correct patient teaching about the IUD. *(262-263)*
    1. "You should not use this contraception if you smoke or are over 35."
    2. "Check for the strings weekly for the first 4 weeks, then monthly."
    3. "Do not use tampons when you have your menstrual period."
    4. "Use another form of contraception for the first month after insertion."

12. Choose the contraceptive method from those listed that provides the best protection against sexually transmitted infections. *(266)*
    1. Female condom
    2. Hormone injection
    3. Intrauterine device
    4. Oral contraceptives

13. When teaching a woman the cervical mucus method to identify ovulation, the nurse teaches her that the normal character of the mucus near ovulation is: *(260)*
    1. slippery and stretchy.
    2. yellowish with a distinct odor.
    3. cloudy and sticky.
    4. thick, sticky, and clear.

14. Appropriate patient teaching following vasectomy is to: *(267)*
    1. apply heat to the operative area for 20 minutes at a time.
    2. abstain from intercourse for at least 6 weeks after the surgery.
    3. limit frequency of sexual intercourse for the first month.
    4. place an ice pack on the operative area to reduce discomfort.

15. A friend tells you that she is "having periods again." She thought she had her last menstrual period 2 years ago. As a nurse, you should advise her that she: *(275)*
    1. is probably having reactivation of estrogens that are causing the bleeding.
    2. should see a physician promptly because this is not an expected occurrence.
    3. may be ovulating again and should use a contraceptive if she does not want to become pregnant.
    4. probably has an infection of her vagina or cervix that should be treated to prevent further infection.

16. "Hot flashes" are probably caused by: *(272)*
    1. anxiety about growing older and one's mortality.
    2. shifts in a woman's fluid and electrolyte balance.
    3. instability of the blood pressure.
    4. reduced estrogen secretion.

17. Choose the correct patient teaching about the drug alendronate (Fosamax). *(273, 275)*
    1. Take food or milk within 30 minutes of the medication.
    2. Wash the nose out with saline 30 minutes after using the spray.
    3. Do not lie down for at least 30 minutes after taking the drug.
    4. Take calcium supplements at the same time as the medication.

18. Stress incontinence is best described as loss of urine: *(276)*
    1. during activities such as laughing or coughing.
    2. when in an anxiety-provoking situation.
    3. when vaginal infection occurs.
    4. during sexual intercourse.

19. What is the usual diagnostic procedure when an ovarian cyst is suspected? *(277)*
    1. Transvaginal ultrasound examination
    2. Bimanual pelvic examination
    3. Laparotomy with biopsy
    4. Magnetic resonance imaging

20. A nursing measure that can improve stress incontinence is to: *(276)*
    1. teach the woman to limit fluid intake to eight glasses of water each day.
    2. advise her to increase her fiber intake with raw vegetables and fruits and whole grains.
    3. encourage weight-bearing exercise at least three times each week.
    4. explain how and when to perform the Kegel exercises.

CHAPTER 12

The Term Newborn

Answer Key: Textbook page references are provided as a guide for answering these questions. A complete answer key was provided for your instructor.

LEARNING ACTIVITIES

1. Why is it important that a governmental agency collect statistical information about births and deaths in the neonatal and infant periods of life? *(279)*

   _____

   _____

   _____

2. Describe each reflex and state the age at which it is expected to disappear. *(280-281)*

Reflex	Description	Age at Disappearance
Moro		
Rooting		
Tonic neck		
Dancing		

3. Normal newborn head circumference ranges from _____ inches to _____ inches, or from _____ cm to _____ cm. *(281)*

4. List two functions of an infant's fontanels. *(281)*

   a. _____

   _____

   b. _____

   _____

5. Describe the following characteristics of the anterior fontanel. *(281-282, Skill 12-1)*

   a. Shape _____

   b. Location (bones) _____

   c. Time of closure _____

6. Describe the following characteristics of the posterior fontanel. *(281, Skill 12-1)*

   a. Shape _____

   b. Location (bones) _____

   c. Time of closure _____

7. Describe the three steps for using a bulb suction to remove a newborn's excess secretions. *(286, Skill 12-2)*

   a. _____

   b. _____

   c. _____

8. Explain the two types of heart murmurs that can be heard in newborns. Indicate which may cause problems. *(287)*

   a. Functional _____

   _____

   b. Organic _____

   _____

9. a. What is a common route for taking a newborn's first temperature? *(287)* _____

   _____

   b. Subsequent temperatures are taken by what route? *(287)* _____

   _____

Student Name _____

    c. What is the correct technique for taking the temperature by each method? *(287)* _____

    _____

    _____

10. State normal ranges for each of these newborn vital signs and signs that the nurse should promptly report. *(287; also Table 9-1, 214, 215, 217)*

Vital Sign	Normal Range (state both Fahrenheit and Centigrade)	Signs to Report (include both rate and character as appropriate)
Temperature		
Pulse		
Respirations		

11. Give the average range for these newborn measurements. *(289)*

    a. Length _____ to _____ inches (_____ to _____ cm)

    b. Weight _____ to _____ pounds (_____ to _____ g)

12. Describe the following normal musculoskeletal assessments for a newborn, including possible deviations from normal. *(288-289)*

    a. Movements _____

    b. Eyes _____

    c. Tremors _____

    d. Muscle tone _____

13. Describe the following characteristics and functions of a newborn infant's kidneys. *(279-280, 289)*

    a. Blood flow _____

    _____

b. Reabsorption functions _____

_____

c. Concentration of urine _____

_____

d. Capacity to handle fluid imbalances _____

_____

14. Expectant parents are attending a prepared childbirth class in which you discuss circumcision. Several ask you if their sons should have the procedure done and another couple said they thought all boys were circumcised. What should you tell these couples about the advantages and disadvantages of circumcision? What should you tell them about circumcision in the Jewish faith? *(289-291)*

a. Advantages _____

_____

b. Disadvantages _____

_____

c. Circumcision in Jewish families _____

_____

15. Explain each of the following aspects of circumcision care in a way you might teach parents. *(291)*

a. Pain relief that may be used _____

_____

b. Comforting _____

_____

c. Maintaining warmth _____

_____

c. Bleeding _____

_____

d. Urination _____

_____

16. Explain the normal occurrences that cause physiologic jaundice. *(291, 294)*

_____

_____

_____

Student Name_____

17. a. Physiologic jaundice appears at about _____ days after birth and lasts for about _____ days. *(291, 294)*

    b. Pathologic jaundice may appear within _____ day(s) after birth. *(291, 294; Chapter 13, 311)*

18. Describe the following typical stools in the newborn, including the time they appear, if applicable. *(294-296)*

    a. Meconium _____

    _____

    b. Transitional stool _____

    _____

    c. Stool of breastfed baby _____

    _____

    d. Stool of formula-fed baby _____

    _____

19. Describe three types of abnormal stools in the newborn. *(296)*

    a. _____

    b. _____

    c. _____

20. Describe stools in constipation. *(296)*

    _____

    _____

21. The newborn's stomach has a capacity of about _____ ml and empties in about _____ hours. *(296)*

22. Why is it important to prevent infection in a newborn and what characteristic of the newborn's response to infection can make it difficult to recognize? *(296-297)*

    _____

    _____

CASE STUDY

1. Sandra and Jim Black, a couple in their mid-20s, have a new son named Justin who is now 16 hours old, weighs 7 pounds, 9 ounces, and is breastfeeding. Sandra wants to go home about 36 hours after birth. Justin will be circumcised (Plastibell) before discharge. Sandra and Jim have no nearby relatives and are the first couple in their circle of friends to have a baby. They have read books on baby care, but are concerned about actually caring for their baby's needs. Sandra and Jim say they need to know "everything."

For each area listed, explain what content you will teach them. How can you encourage the parents to participate in each topic so they will feel more secure? How will you incorporate information they may have read in books? You are encouraged to use any of your facility's teaching materials as you complete this case study.

a. Safety
b. Using bulb syringe
c. Taking their baby's temperature
d. Maintaining an optimal body temperature

2. Because Justin will be discharged soon after being circumcised, what should you teach the parents about care and observation for complications? What actions may comfort him?

APPLYING KNOWLEDGE

1. Assist with admitting newborns. Administer prophylactic eye care and vitamin K injections. What initial and ongoing cord care does your facility use and with what frequency? Does your facility offer the first hepatitis B immunization with newborn care? Do parents sign a consent form for any of these procedures? Which one(s)?

2. Does your facility use an instrument to check bilirubin levels in the newborn's skin? Describe how the nurse arrives at the most accurate bilirubin level with the instrument and how that level is documented.

3. Observe newborns in the nursery for characteristics listed in the textbook. Distinguish between normal characteristics and those that may indicate a problem. What action is taken for deviations from normal?

4. Observe a circumcision. What type of circumcision is most common in your hospital? Observe newborns after circumcision for bleeding and urination.

5. Does your hospital have a standard infant care teaching plan for new parents? If so, what does the plan include? Observe how different staff nurses incorporate parent teaching into their care of mothers and babies. How have short stays influenced parent teaching?

6. A baby is coming to the office for a checkup at 1 week of age. He weighed 8 pounds, 6 ounces at birth. He now weighs 7 pounds, 7 ounces. Has the baby's weight loss been within normal limits or is it excessive? Justify your answer.

REVIEW QUESTIONS

1. Which reflex shows the baby's reaction to sudden movement by drawing up the legs, extending the arms, then folding the arms across the chest with the fingers open? *(280)*
   1. Dancing
   2. Moro
   3. Rooting
   4. Grasp

2. When teaching a mother how to nurse her baby, how should you explain the baby's rooting reflex? The rooting reflex: *(280)*
   1. shows equality of function on each side of the mouth.
   2. helps the baby keep mucus or milk from being inhaled during breathing.
   3. suggests that the baby is full as he or she turns away from the breast.
   4. is the baby's way of seeking her nipple to obtain milk when hungry.

Student Name_____

3. In the birthing room, a first-time father asks the nurse why the baby's head is "long and pointy." The nurse should respond: *(281)*
    1. "The head changes shape so it can pass through the mother's pelvis during birth."
    2. "Fluid builds up within the head before and during birth; it will go away in a few days."
    3. "Labor causes slight bleeding into the space between the skull bones and their covering."
    4. "We will notify the pediatrician, who will probably order an MRI of the baby's head."

4. Visually, babies prefer: *(281)*
    1. geometric objects.
    2. soft or pastel colors.
    3. the human face.
    4. stationary objects.

5. The correct way to suction a baby's mouth with a bulb syringe is to: *(286)*
    1. compress the bulb, place the tip in the side of the mouth, then release the bulb.
    2. place the tip in the side of the mouth, compress the bulb, then release the bulb.
    3. compress the bulb, place the tip in the center of the mouth, then release the bulb.
    4. place the tip in the center of the mouth, compress the bulb, then release the bulb.

6. When admitted to the nursery, a baby's initial rectal temperature is 96.6° F (35.8° C). Choose the most appropriate nursing response for this assessment. *(287-288)*
    1. Chart the expected temperature and continue doing other admission assessments and measurements.
    2. Keep the baby in a radiant warmer during admission and recheck the temperature in 30 minutes.
    3. Remove blankets and sources of added heat from the baby.
    4. Recheck the temperature in 30 minutes to verify accuracy.

7. One hour after a Plastibell circumcision, the nurse notes a small amount of blood oozing from the area. Which is the appropriate initial nursing response to this observation? *(291)*
    1. Continue to observe for increased bleeding.
    2. Apply pressure with a gauze pad and gloved fingers.
    3. Call the physician who performed the procedure.
    4. Wrap petroleum jelly gauze around the penis.

8. A new mother asks why her 2-day-old baby's skin appears slightly yellow. Which is the best nursing response to explain the cause of this skin color? *(291, 294)*
    1. Small blood vessels are broken during labor, releasing waste products into the blood.
    2. The baby's digestive tract is immature and cannot yet excrete bilirubin effectively.
    3. Skin color changes slightly during the first few weeks until the permanent color is evident.
    4. Excess blood cells are being broken down rapidly because the baby is now breathing air.

9. New parents should be taught to clean their baby's ears by: *(284)*
    1. moistening a cotton-tipped applicator with water and rotating it in the ear canal.
    2. gently instilling a small amount of warm water into the ear with a bulb syringe.
    3. applying baby oil to a rolled piece of cotton and inserting it into the ear.
    4. wiping the outside with a cotton ball that is moistened with water.

10. A small area of a term infant's abdominal skin remains distorted when pinched gently. This assessment suggests: *(291)*
    1. poor hydration.
    2. postbirth edema.
    3. excessive intake of breast milk or formula.
    4. inadequate vernix during the prenatal period.

11. What should the parents be taught about caring for the umbilical cord? *(294)*
    1. Bathe the baby in a small basin to cleanse the cord on all surfaces.
    2. A sponge bath is easy and allows the cord to remain dry until healed.
    3. Use an oil-based cleanser to speed healing of the baby's cord site.
    4. Baths are not needed until the cord site has healed to reduce infection.

12. An infant has a small laceration on the forehead when delivered by cesarean. Brief finger pressure in the operating room stopped the bleeding and the physician does not need to suture the laceration. The nurse should primarily observe for what other complication related to the baby's laceration? *(296-297)*
    1. Anemia, possibly manifested by pallor and tachycardia
    2. Hypothermia due to delay of placement in a warmer
    3. Excessive erythrocyte destruction and early jaundice
    4. Infection limited to the site or possibly generalized

13. A newborn has a heelstick for studies. The mother is concerned because the baby is crying loudly. The best response of the nurse is: *(291)*
    1. "That's the only way the baby can communicate with us."
    2. "Hold the baby close and comfort him by gentle rocking."
    3. "Babies cannot feel pain because they are immature."
    4. "The baby will only cry for a few minutes at most."

14. How should the nurse respond to acrocyanosis in a 12-hour-old infant? *(291)*
    1. Administer oxygen through an infant-sized mask.
    2. Apply heat with an incubator or radiant warmer.
    3. Assess the pulse and respirations for abnormal rates.
    4. Continue routine newborn nursing observations.

15. Which is an abnormal clinic assessment for a Latino boy at 1 week of age? Birth weight was 8 pounds, 5 ounces (3772 g); vital signs at hospital discharge time were: T 98.4° F (axillary); P 142; R 40. There were no complications during pregnancy. *(289)*
    1. The infant weighs 7 pounds, 5 ounces (3318 g).
    2. The apical pulse is 130 bpm and slightly irregular.
    3. The infant has bluish areas on the lower back.
    4. The infant has tiny white raised papules on the nose.

16. A new mother asks why her term newborn sometimes "shakes" when he cries. Choose the best nursing response. *(284, 289)*
    1. "Why not ask the baby's doctor about this when she makes rounds?"
    2. "The baby is easily upset and waves his arms to show his irritation."
    3. "An infant's muscles are too weak to move steadily."
    4. "This is a normal newborn behavior during crying."

17. A term newborn should pass the first meconium stool no later than how many hours after birth? *(294)*
    1. 6
    2. 12
    3. 24
    4. 36

Student Name_____

18. A new mother is concerned because her 3-day-old daughter has a slightly blood-tinged vaginal mucus discharge. How should the nurse respond to this mother's concern? *(291)*
    1. "The baby could have a minor abnormality in her vagina."
    2. "Has there been any kind of injury to this area?"
    3. "Effects of your pregnancy hormones cause this response."
    4. "This should be reported to the doctor right away."

19. The nurse should teach parents to avoid using baby powder because it: *(294)*
    1. irritates the newborn's respiratory tract.
    2. may cause allergies in the newborn.
    3. is difficult to remove during a bath.
    4. dries the skin of the axillae and groin.

20. An infant looks at her mother and remains quiet when the mother sings to her in soft, high-pitched tones. This is an example of: *(284)*
    1. a sign of impaired hearing.
    2. the quiet alert state of reactivity.
    3. a need for reduced stimulation.
    4. limited ability to respond to adults.

CROSSWORD PUZZLE

Across

2. First stool *(294)*
4. Fetal skin protectant from watery environment *(291)*
9. Edema of the scalp *(Figure 12-5, 281, 283)*
10. Soft area at intersection of skull bones *(281-282)*
13. White dots on the palate with the appearance of pearls *(291)*
15. Bluish color of the hands and feet *(287)*
16. Small white bumps, usually on the nose or chin *(291)*

Down

1. Failure of the testes to descend into the scrotum *(289)*
2. Bluish spots or discolorations of the skin, usually in dark-skinned babies *(291)*
3. Shaping of the head from pressure during birth *(281)*
5. Removal of the foreskin of the penis *(289)*
6. Collection of blood beneath the periosteum of the skull *(281)*
7. Urethral opening on the underside of penis *(289)*
8. Fine hair covering the body *(291)*
11. Term used to describe tissue elasticity *(291)*
12. Topical anesthetic used for pain relief during circumcision *(285, 290, Figure 12-12)*
14. "Bites" that are not really bites, but reddish areas on the back of the neck and eyelids. *(291)*

CHAPTER 13

Student Name _____

Preterm and Postterm Newborns

Answer Key: Textbook page references are provided as a guide for answering these questions. A complete answer key was provided for your instructor.

LEARNING ACTIVITIES

1. Match the terms in the left column with their definitions on the right (a–p).

_____ Apnea *(308)*	a. Provision of full nutrition by the parenteral (IV) route
_____ Ballard *(304-306)*	b. Length of time spent in the uterus
_____ Bradycardia *(308)*	c. Cessation of breathing for 20 seconds or more
_____ Bronchopulmonary dysplasia *(307)*	d. Lung secretion that facilitates oxygen exchange
_____ Circadian rhythm *(315)*	e. Nervous system damage caused by high levels of bilirubin in the blood
_____ Gestational age *(304)*	f. Method of estimating newborn maturity by physical and neurological characteristics
_____ Hypoglycemia *(309)*	g. Heart rate lower than 100 bpm in the newborn
_____ Kangaroo care *(312, 314)*	h. Generalized infection
_____ Kernicterus *(311)*	i. Low blood glucose (blood sugar) level
_____ Neutral thermal environment *(312)*	j. Control of temperature, air, surface temperature, and humidity to minimize an infant's oxygen consumption
_____ Preterm gestation *(304)*	k. Less than 38 weeks of gestation
_____ Postterm gestation *(304)*	l. 38 to 42 weeks of gestation
_____ Sepsis *(308)*	m. More than 42 weeks of gestation
_____ Surfactant *(305)*	n. Warming an infant by skin-to-skin contact
_____ Term gestation *(304)*	o. Sleep pattern
_____ Total parenteral nutrition *(315)*	p. Condition that may cause an infant to have a prolonged dependence on a ventilator

2. Describe the following typical physical characteristics of a preterm infant's appearance. *(305)*

   a. Skin _____

   b. Superficial veins _____

   c. Subcutaneous fat _____

    d. Lanugo _____

    e. Vernix caseosa _____

    f. Sole creases _____

    g. Abdomen _____

    h. Nails _____

    i. Genitalia _____

3. a. Respiratory distress syndrome (RDS) is associated with an inadequate quantity of _____ in the lungs. *(305-308)*

    b. At what gestational age is an infant expected to have an adequate quantity of this substance? *(305-308)*

    _____

    c. If an infant is born before the gestational age in 3 b, what is the usual therapy? *(305-308)*

    _____

4. If preterm birth appears inevitable, what drug for the mother should the nurse anticipate before birth? *(306)*

    _____

5. List two signs that may accompany apnea. *(308)*

    a. _____

    b. _____

6. List seven factors that make the preterm infant more vulnerable to loss of body heat than a term infant. *(308-309)*

    a. _____

    b. _____

    c. _____

    d. _____

    e. _____

    f. _____

    g. _____

7. a. Hypoglycemia in the infant is defined as a plasma level of glucose lower than _____ mg/dl. *(309)*

    b. List two reasons why a preterm infant is prone to hypoglycemia. *(309)*

    _____

    _____

Student Name_____

8. What two factors predispose a preterm infant to bleeding? *(309)*

   a. _____

   b. _____

9. Describe five factors that impair the preterm infant's nutritional function. *(310)*

   a. _____

   b. _____

   c. _____

   d. _____

   e. _____

10. a. What is the pathology of necrotizing enterocolitis (NEC)? *(311)*

    _____

    _____

    b. List signs that an infant may have NEC. *(311)*

    _____

    _____

11. a. Pathologic jaundice may appear within _____ (time) and/or may increase at a rate greater than _____/24 hours. *(291,294; 311)*

    b. Breast milk jaundice usually appears at _____ (time) and peaks _____ to _____ days after birth. *(291,294; 311)*

    c. Explain why the infant with breast milk jaundice may receive formula. How long is formula substituted for this infant? *(291,294; 311)*

    _____

    _____

    _____

12. The ideal milk for the preterm infant is _____ milk. *(312)*

13. List three methods by which the preterm infant can receive nourishment. *(312, 315)*

    a. _____

    b. _____

    c. _____

14. a. The two usual positions for the preterm infant are _____ or _____ _____. *(315)*

b. What two alternate positions may be used for the preterm infant and why? *(315)*

_____

_____

15. List seven problems that are associated with caring for a postterm newborn. *(316-317)*

a. _____

b. _____

c. _____

d. _____

e. _____

f. _____

g. _____

16. Describe the following typical physical characteristics of the postterm newborn. *(316-317)*

a. General body appearance _____

_____

b. Presence of lanugo _____

_____

c. Presence of vernix caseosa _____

_____

d. Skin appearance _____

_____

THINKING CRITICALLY

1. A friend had her baby at 32 weeks gestation 6 months ago. She confides that she is afraid her baby is not normal because he does not do the same things her first baby (born at term) did at 6 months old. What can you tell your friend to reassure her?

Student Name_____

APPLYING KNOWLEDGE

1. Observe newborns of different gestational ages in your clinical facility. Identify differences in these characteristics. Determine whether the mother's "due date" correlates with the physical characteristics you see. Do you note any differences if an infant is delivered by scheduled induction or cesarean?
   a. Head and body hair
   b. Body posture and muscle tone
   c. Stiffness of ear cartilage
   d. Amount of breast tissue
   e. Appearance of genitalia
   f. Number and depth of sole creases

2. Observe different methods of feeding preterm infants. What precautions are taken to ensure that the baby receives adequate nutrition without overload?

3. If your facility does not routinely care for sick newborns, does it have arrangements with a larger hospital to transport these babies to a special care nursery? What is involved in transporting a sick baby? When do most newborns return to the original facility or are they usually discharged by the special care nursery in the larger hospital?

4. How does your facility foster parent-infant bonding when an infant is sick or preterm? Is kangaroo care used? Are facilities available for parents of the infant transported a long distance, such as Ronald McDonald houses?

5. Look up facility policies that relate to neonatal jaundice. Do specific definitions describe bilirubin levels and treatment for physiologic, pathologic, and breast milk jaundice?

REVIEW QUESTIONS

1. Which of the following physical characteristics should make the nurse think an infant's gestational age may be preterm? *(306)*
   1. Square window sign assessed at 0 degrees
   2. Small amount of lanugo and vernix present
   3. Labia majora cover labia minora of the female
   4. Superficial scalp and abdominal veins easily seen

2. Gestational age is best determined with: *(304-305)*
   1. weight of the infant at birth.
   2. stability of the blood glucose level.
   3. the age at which the infant reaches developmental milestones.
   4. assessment of physical and neurological characteristics.

3. A preterm infant is subject to hypothermia because the: *(308-309)*
   1. muscle activity is large related to the calories consumed.
   2. relatively large body surface area allows heat to escape.
   3. sweat glands are overactive, allowing evaporative cooling.
   4. fat stores insulate the infant from radiant heater warmth.

4. Choose the normal blood glucose level for a preterm infant. *(309)*
   1. 28 mg/dl
   2. 39 mg/dl
   3. 55 mg/dl
   4. 150 mg/dl

5. The nurse must handle the preterm infant gently because capillaries are: *(309)*
   1. not developed in all areas of the brain.
   2. likely to develop microscopic clots.
   3. sensitive to high levels of clotting factors.
   4. fragile and prone to bleed spontaneously.

6. The advantage of radiant heaters in the care of preterm infants is that they: *(312)*
   1. cannot cause excessive body temperature.
   2. maintain warmth with easy caregiver access.
   3. reduce drying and cracking of the skin.
   4. improve balance of fluids and electrolytes.

7. The ideal feeding for most preterm newborns is: *(312)*
   1. glucose water until the risk for necrotizing enterocolitis diminishes.
   2. breast milk given by suckling, bottle, or gavage.
   3. special commercial formula for preterm babies.
   4. total parenteral nutrition to meet all the infant's nutritional needs.

8. An infant is brought to the newborn nursery. The gestation stated on the chart is 39 weeks. The nurse doing the initial assessment notes that the infant has peeling skin and a long, thin appearance. What is the probable reason for the infant's appearance? *(316-317)*
   1. The mother did not get adequate nutrients throughout pregnancy.
   2. Intrauterine infection depleted subcutaneous fat stores.
   3. The actual gestational age may be greater than 42 weeks.
   4. Reduced production of glucose before birth caused weight loss.

9. A mother gives birth to a preterm infant at 30 weeks gestation. When visiting the baby in the intensive care unit, she seems interested in the baby, but sits and watches everything the nurse does for her baby. Which is the most appropriate nursing intervention to promote mother-infant attachment? *(316)*
   1. Invite her to provide simple care to her infant.
   2. Reassure her that she can hold the baby soon.
   3. Stress the importance of frequent visits to the nursery.
   4. Demonstrate the skills she will need for home care.

10. Which nursing assessment best suggests respiratory distress syndrome? *(305-306)*
    1. Apical heart rate 144/min; bluish hands and feet
    2. Grunting, respiratory rate of 65/min, nasal flaring
    3. Protruding abdomen, irregular respirations
    4. Weak movements, lies with extended posture

11. The alarm on an apnea monitor for a preterm infant sounds. The infant is asleep, the skin color is pink, and the heart rate is 130–135/min. The most appropriate initial nursing response is to: *(308)*
    1. contact the physician for orders.
    2. gently rub the infant's back.
    3. give oxygen with an Ambu bag.
    4. suction the infant with a bulb syringe.

Student Name_____

12. A key nursing intervention to prevent retinopathy of prematurity is to: *(309-310; Skill 13-1)*
    1. provide feedings as early as possible after birth.
    2. perform care to avoid moving the infant more than necessary.
    3. eliminate potential sources of infection from the environment.
    4. monitor the infant's blood oxygen levels.

13. Most problems of the postterm infant result from: *(316-317)*
    1. decreased functioning of the placenta.
    2. reduced blood clotting factors.
    3. increased susceptibility to infection.
    4. thicker subcutaneous fat deposits.

14. Choose the bilirubin level or levels that should be reported to the physician for an infant of 38 weeks gestation. *(311)*
    1. 4 mg/dl at 18 hours after birth; 12 mg prior to discharge at 36 hours
    2. 6 mg/dl at 24 hours after birth; sclerae and face are yellowish
    3. 9 mg/dl prior to hospital discharge at 48 hours after birth
    4. 6 mg/dl at 24 hours after birth; infant is breastfeeding well

Student Name _____

CHAPTER 14

The Newborn with a Congenital Malformation

Answer Key: Textbook page references are provided as a guide for answering these questions. A complete answer key was provided for your instructor.

LEARNING ACTIVITIES

1. Match the terms in the left column with their definitions on the right (a–p).

   _____ Cheiloplasty *(326)*

   _____ Habilitation *(323)*

   _____ Hydrocephalus *(320)*

   _____ Hyperbilirubinemia *(337)*

   _____ Kernicterus *(337)*

   _____ Macrosomia *(343)*

   _____ Meningocele *(323)*

   _____ Myelodysplasia *(323)*

   _____ Meningomyelocele *(323)*

   _____ Neonatal abstinence syndrome *(342)*

   _____ Ortolani's sign *(329)*

   _____ Pavlik harness *(329)*

   _____ Simian crease *(334)*

   _____ Subluxation *(329)*

   _____ Transillumination *(321)*

   _____ Trisomy *(334)*

   a. Inspection of a cavity or organ by passing a light through its walls
   b. Suggests developmental hip dysplasia
   c. Teaching a skill to a child who is handicapped from birth
   d. Maintains hip abduction in the treatment of developmental hip dysplasia
   e. Single transverse line across the palm
   f. Brain damage due to accumulation of bilirubin in the brain tissue
   g. Large fetal or newborn body size
   h. Surgical repair of a cleft lip
   i. Partial displacement of the head of the femur from the acetabulum
   j. Excess blood levels of bilirubin
   k. Presence of one extra chromosome in a body cell
   l. Group of malformations of the spinal cord
   m. Accumulation of cerebrospinal fluid within the brain's ventricles
   n. Form of spina bifida in which portions of the membranes and cerebrospinal fluid are contained in a cystic mass
   o. Form of spina bifida that consists of protrusion of a saclike cyst containing meninges, spinal fluid, and a portion of the spinal cord with its nerves
   p. Fetal exposure to maternal drugs that cause dependence

2. List five classes of congenital anomalies that may occur in the neonate. Give one or more examples of each. *(320)*

   a. _____

   b. _____

   c. _____

   d. _____

   e. _____

3. List the two classifications of hydrocephalus and describe features of each. *(320-321)*

   a. _____

   _____

   b. _____

   _____

4. List two possible complications of shunts for treatment of hydrocephalus. *(321)*

   a. _____

   b. _____

5. Why is it essential to frequently change position if an infant has an enlarged head due to hydrocephalus but has not yet had a shunt? *(321-322)*

   _____

   _____

6. List signs of the two primary complications that may occur after shunt placement for hydrocephalus. *(322)*

   a. Infection of the shunt _____

   _____

   b. Increased intracranial pressure _____

   _____

7. What is the current recommendation for all women related to prevention of neural tube defects such as meningomyelocele? *(323)*

   _____

   _____

Student Name_____

8. Describe nursing observations and care for the newborn with spina bifida in each of the following areas. *(323-326)*

   a. Care of the sac before surgical repair _____

   _____

   b. Extremities _____

   _____

   c. Head _____

   _____

   d. Bowel and bladder function _____

   _____

   e. Latex allergy _____

   _____

9. What are the positioning options the nurse may use for a child with a myelocele or meningomyelocele before surgical repair? *(325)*

   _____

   _____

10. Describe postoperative nursing care for the child with a cleft lip and/or palate repair. *(326-327)*

   a. Preventing injury to the operative site _____

   _____

   b. Positioning _____

   _____

   c. Prevention of infection _____

   _____

   d. Emotional care _____

   _____

   e. Pain relief _____

   _____

11. Describe three ways of treating clubfoot. *(328)*

   a. _____

   b. _____

   c. _____

12. Describe nursing care of the child who has a cast on both legs. *(328)*

_____

_____

_____

_____

13. List four signs of developmental hip dysplasia in the infant. *(329)*

    a. _____

    _____

    b. _____

    _____

    c. _____

    _____

    d. _____

    _____

14. What procedure should the nurse use to turn a child in a body cast (spica)? *(330-332, Skill 14-1)*

_____

_____

_____

_____

_____

_____

15. a. Explain how and when the nurse will screen a newborn for phenylketonuria (PKU). *(332-333)*

    _____

    _____

    _____

    b. An infant's PKU screening is positive. What confirmation test is done for positive results on a screening test? *(332-333)*

    _____

    _____

Student Name _____

16. Describe the manifestations of the listed inborn errors of metabolism, how they are diagnosed, and their treatment. *(333-334)*

    a.   Maple syrup urine disease _____

    _____

    _____

    b.   Galactosemia _____

    _____

    _____

17. Describe physical and developmental characteristics that may be seen in a child with Down syndrome. *(334-336)*

    a.   Facial features _____

    _____

    b.   Hands and feet _____

    _____

    c.   Musculoskeletal characteristics _____

    _____

    d.   Internal abnormalities _____

    _____

    e.   Physical and intellectual development _____

    _____

18. Parents of children born with Down syndrome have special needs. Give examples of how the nurse could help parents meet these needs. *(334-336)*

    a.   Resistance to infection _____

    _____

    b.   Hypotonic muscles and loose joints _____

    _____

    c.   Constipation _____

    _____

    d.   Grieving _____

    _____

19. Describe occurrences in the pathophysiology of erythroblastosis fetalis. *(336-337)*

_____

_____

20. a. What drug can prevent development of erythroblastosis fetalis and who (mother or infant) should receive it? *(336-338)*

_____

_____

    b. List five circumstances in which the drug is indicated. *(336-338)*

       (1)_____

       (2)_____

       (3)_____

       (4)_____

       (5)_____

21. Explain related nursing care in each of the following areas if an infant must receive phototherapy in an incubator rather than with a fiberoptic pad or blanket. *(337-341, Nursing Care Plan 14-2)*

    a. Eye protection _____

_____

    b. Protection of ovaries or testes _____

_____

    c. Potential dehydration _____

_____

22. Intracranial hemorrhage around the time of birth is usually caused by _____ or _____. *(341-342)*

23. List signs that should make the nurse suspect that a newborn has had an intracranial hemorrhage. *(341)*

_____

_____

_____

_____

24. What are two possible permanent effects of an intracranial hemorrhage? *(341)*

    a. _____

    b. _____

Student Name _____

25. a. What causes the infants of some diabetic mothers to be larger than expected for their gestational age? *(343)*

_____

_____

b. What are other possible outcomes for the infant when the woman has diabetes during pregnancy? *(343)*

_____

_____

c. What blood test should the nurse expect to perform when an infant is born to a diabetic mother? What is the normal level for a newborn? *(343)*

_____

_____

CASE STUDIES

1. A newborn who has a meningomyelocele has paralysis of the legs and is dribbling urine and stool.
   a. Identify four nursing concerns for the nurse caring for the baby.
   b. What can the nurse tell the infant's parents about the dribbling of urine and oozing of stool as it relates to skin care and future control of these functions?
   c. How should the nurse involve the parents in the infant's care in the newborn nursery?
   d. What related problems should the nurse observe for in this infant? What signs should make the nurse suspect that the problems have developed?

2. Dianna, 4 months old, is brought to the hospital by her mother because she had a seizure this morning. The admission physical exam shows an irritable, thin, lethargic child who the mother says has been vomiting the small amount of formula she would eat. Her height and weight measurements are below normal and her head circumference is slightly larger than normal. Dianna has not had any health care since her birth in a distant city. The admitting diagnosis is suspected hydrocephalus.
   a. Is Dianna exhibiting any signs of increased intracranial pressure? List observations that would support your conclusion.
   b. List diagnostic tests that may be done to confirm this diagnosis.
   c. What nursing measures should the nurse take to promote skin integrity?
   d. How should the nurse position Dianna during and after feedings?

APPLYING KNOWLEDGE

1. If you have a pediatric patient with Down syndrome (trisomy 21), compare the development of gross and fine motor abilities of the child with those of a child of the same approximate age who does not have Down syndrome. Has the child with Down syndrome had any of the associated problems such as respiratory infections, ear infections, or heart defects?

2. While in the clinical area, care for a child or adult who has Down syndrome. If you have a friend or family member with Down syndrome, tell your classmates what you have learned over time.

3. Observe the repair of a cleft lip or cleft palate. If unable to observe an existing cleft or its repair, observe the results of a repair from a future patient if possible.

4. Care for an infant receiving phototherapy with a fiberoptic pad or blanket. What is the most likely cause for the hyperbilirubinemia in this child? Are term infants discharged from your facility for home phototherapy? What procedures are followed for starting and follow-up of home phototherapy? Is exposure to natural light utilized to reduce bilirubin levels?

5. Give $Rh_o(D)$ immune globulin (RhoGAM) under instructor supervision. Why is this patient having the medication at this time?

REVIEW QUESTIONS

1. A sign that should make the nurse suspect hydrocephalus in the newborn is: *(321)*
   1. inability to sleep between feedings.
   2. a patch of hair on the lower back.
   3. axillary temperature of 37.8° C (100° F).
   4. an enlarged fontanel or cranial sutures.

2. Expected treatment for hydrocephalus is: *(321)*
   1. placement of a shunt.
   2. incision and draining.
   3. oral liquid diuretics.
   4. intravenous analgesics.

3. Vital sign changes when an infant has increased intracranial pressure include: *(322)*
   1. increased blood pressure and pulse, hyperventilation.
   2. decreased blood pressure, pulse, and respirations.
   3. decreased blood pressure and respirations, increased pulse.
   4. increased blood pressure, decreased pulse and respirations.

4. Before surgical repair, the usual position of a newborn with a meningomyelocele is: *(325)*
   1. side-lying with the head slightly below the level of the heart.
   2. prone, maintaining abduction with a pad between the legs.
   3. supine with the crib flat to stabilize blood pressure.
   4. supine with the legs widely abducted and thighs flexed.

5. Which of the following nursing measures is appropriate for a 2-week-old infant who has a new cleft lip repair? *(326-327)*
   1. Position on the abdomen or side
   2. Place in a car seat after each feeding
   3. Provide a premature-sized pacifier
   4. Limit visitors to immediate family

6. A priority of postoperative nursing care for a 9-month-old infant who has cleft palate repair is: *(327)*
   1. referral to a parent support group.
   2. adequate nutrition.
   3. keeping an intravenous line open.
   4. continuous sedation.

Student Name _____

7. Appropriate care related to a new plaster cast for correction of clubfoot in the newborn is to: *(328)*
   1. keep the infant snugly wrapped until the cast is dry to prevent hypothermia.
   2. sprinkle powder into the dry cast to reduce skin irritation at the edges of the cast.
   3. position with the feet lower than the level of the heart until the cast is dry.
   4. observe the toes for pallor, cyanosis, reduced capillary refill, or cold temperature.

8. When checking range of motion of an infant, what sign suggests developmental hip dysplasia? *(330-331)*
   1. Reduced thigh abduction
   2. Full abduction and adduction
   3. Equal gluteal creases in the back
   4. Limited flexion of one knee

9. A 2-week-old infant will be fitted with a Pavlik harness as treatment for developmental hip dysplasia. The mother asks the nurse about the harness and how it will help her baby. To reinforce the physician's explanation, the nurse should teach the mother that: *(329-330)*
   1. keeping the hip bone within the hip socket helps the socket to become deeper.
   2. the infant cannot have surgery for the condition until he is at least 8 weeks old.
   3. the longer leg gradually becomes shorter to equalize the leg lengths before walking.
   4. time spent in a cast is reduced if the baby is treated with a harness for a few weeks.

10. The nurse should suspect intracranial hemorrhage in a newborn because: *(341)*
    1. the fontanel is of normal size but depressed.
    2. muscle tone has become poor since birth.
    3. the infant seems to be hungry much of the time.
    4. both pupils are small and react to light when checked.

11. The child with PKU must be on a diet that is: *(332-333)*
    1. low in fatty acids to promote intellectual development.
    2. high in soluble fiber to reduce constipation.
    3. low in phenylalanine to limit buildup of the protein.
    4. fluid-restricted to reduce the wastes delivered to the kidneys.

12. Early identification of galactosemia is required to prevent: *(333)*
    1. depletion of specific amino acids.
    2. liver damage, cataracts, and mental retardation.
    3. protein deposits in the adrenal glands and kidneys.
    4. limitation of normal growth in height.

13. Appropriate nursing care for parents immediately after the birth of a baby who has characteristics typical of Down syndrome should include: *(334)*
    1. reassuring them that future babies are unlikely to have this problem.
    2. keeping the infant in the nursery until a definitive diagnosis is made.
    3. spending time with them so they can best verbalize their concerns.
    4. teaching them about lifelong nutritional care the baby will need.

14. Parent-infant bonding in an infant with a meningomyelocele prior to repair can be enhanced by: *(326)*
    1. encouraging the parents to talk to and touch the baby.
    2. having the parents change the baby's diaper.
    3. encouraging the parents to hold the baby near their skin.
    4. helping a parent give the baby an admission bath.

15. The mother of a 2-week-old infant who is going to have a cleft lip repair asks if she will be able to hold her baby after surgery. The nurse should reply: *(326)*
    1. "The baby can be held when she no longer needs the restraints."
    2. "The baby cannot be held but you can talk to her and stroke her."
    3. "Holding your baby helps to keep her content."
    4. "You should hold your baby only during feedings."

16. An Rh-negative woman who gives birth to an Rh-positive infant should receive $Rh_o(D)$ immune globulin (RhoGAM) no later than _____ hours after birth. *(336-337)*
    1. 4–8
    2. 16
    3. 24–36
    4. 72

17. Expected advice for the woman with PKU who is considering pregnancy is to eat a daily diet that: *(333)*
    1. contains additional high-fiber foods.
    2. contains adequate dairy products.
    3. provides added amounts of leucine.
    4. has low quantities of phenylalanine.

18. The infant with Down syndrome is at increased risk for developing: *(334)*
    1. urinary tract infections.
    2. respiratory infections.
    3. kidney infections.
    4. meningitis.

19. What complication is more likely for an infant of a diabetic mother within the first few hours after birth? *(343)*
    1. Intracranial hemorrhage
    2. Hyperactive reflexes
    3. Excessive urination
    4. Low blood glucose levels

20. Why might an infant of a diabetic mother be small for gestational age (SGA)? *(343)*
    1. The placenta did not receive adequate perfusion during pregnancy.
    2. The fetus had episodes of hypoglycemia when the mother took insulin.
    3. The fetal pancreas does not make insulin if the mother takes insulin.
    4. The mother's diabetes causes small areas of bleeding in the placenta.

21. Meconium aspiration syndrome may be prevented by: *(342)*
    1. stimulating the infant to breathe as soon as delivery is complete.
    2. reducing meconium in amniotic fluid before birth by amnioinfusion.
    3. intubating the infant immediately after birth for ventilation.
    4. promoting adequate infant oxygenation with an apnea monitor.

CHAPTER 15

An Overview of Growth, Development, and Nutrition

Answer Key: Textbook page references are provided as a guide for answering these questions. A complete answer key was provided for your instructor.

LEARNING ACTIVITIES

1. Match the terms in the left column with their definitions on the right (a–f).

    _____ Cephalocaudal *(348)*
    _____ Development *(348)*
    _____ Growth *(348)*
    _____ Maturation *(348)*
    _____ Parallel play *(378)*
    _____ Proximodistal *(348)*

    a. Progressive increase in physical size
    b. Progressive increase in body function
    c. Total way a person grows and develops, dictated by inheritance
    d. Head-to-toe developmental pattern
    e. Central-to-peripheral developmental pattern
    f. Activity alongside another child or children

Answer as either true (T) or false (F).

2. Children grow at a steady rate and in an orderly process. *(345)* _____

3. Development proceeds from simple to complex. *(345)* _____

4. List the age range (in months or years) of each of the following stages. *(347)*

    a. Fetus _____

    b. Newborn _____

    c. Infant _____

    d. Toddler _____

    e. Preschool child _____

    f. School-age child _____

    g. Adolescent _____

5. Give a specific example of each type of developmental pattern. *(348)*

   a. Cephalocaudal _____

   b. Proximodistal _____

6. What are the two most rapid periods of growth after birth? *(348)*

   a. _____

   b. _____

7. Birth weight usually _____ by 6 months of age and _____ by 1 year. *(348)*

8. How does the percentage of body fluid change as the infant matures to adulthood? Why is it important for the nurse to know this? *(348)*

   _____

   _____

   _____

   _____

9. Why would a burn chart for calculating percentage of injured body surface area for an adult be inappropriate for a child with burns? *(348)*

   _____

   _____

   _____

10. Why are ear infections more common in young children? *(348)*

    _____

    _____

    _____

    _____

11. What factors contribute to the development of physiologic anemia in a 3-month-old infant? *(349)*

    _____

    _____

12. Infants are susceptible to dehydration because _____

    _____. *(349)*

Student Name _____

13. The Denver II assesses the _____ status of children from birth to 6 years of age in the following four categories: *(352)*

    a. _____

    b. _____

    c. _____

    d. _____

Answer as either true (T) or false (F).

14. The Denver II is an intelligence test. *(352)* _____

15. A low score on the Denver II indicates that a child has a developmental delay. *(352)* _____

16. A dysfunctional family implies its members are not loving and caring. *(354)* _____

17. List five factors that can influence a child's growth and development. *(353)*

    a. _____

    b. _____

    c. _____

    d. _____

    e. _____

18. How can physical illness affect a child's growth and development? *(353)*

    _____

19. List the components of the family APGAR. *(354)*

    A _____

    P _____

    G _____

    A _____

    R _____

20. Define *systems theory*. *(355)*

    _____

    _____

    _____

21. Match the following behaviors with the correct stages of Piaget's theory of cognitive development (a–d).

   _____   Sensorimotor *(361)*
   _____   Preoperational *(361)*
   _____   Concrete operations *(361)*
   _____   Formal operations *(361)*

   a. Progresses from reflexes to intentional interaction with the environment
   b. Develops ability for hypothetical and abstract thought
   c. Views the world egocentrically
   d. Reasoning becomes logical; understands cause and effect

22. Describe the moral development of a 5-year-old child. *(361)*

   _____

   _____

   _____

23. How can parents' knowledge of growth and development help prevent accidents in children? *(362)*

   _____

   _____

   _____

   _____

24. Why might a child who eats a vegetarian diet be anemic? *(366)*

   _____

   _____

   _____

   _____

25. What is the food of choice for the first 6 months to 1 year of life? *(369)*_____

   _____

26. Why are restrictive diets not recommended for infants and young children? *(369)*

   _____

27. The first solid food introduced to infants is usually _____. *(370)*

28. Solids foods are introduced into the infant's diet at what age? *(371)*_____

29. What is the earliest age that a child should begin whole milk? *(372)* _____

30. One guideline for determining the appropriate amount of food to feed to children is _____ tablespoon(s) of food for each year of age. *(373)*

31. Primary dentition is completed by _____. *(374)*

32. The first primary teeth erupt at _____ months. *(375)*

Student Name_____

Answer as either true (T) or false (F).

33. Carbohydrate consumption is the most important dietary consideration for dental health. *(376)* _____

34. The child should be encouraged to brush his or her teeth after eating sticky foods. *(376)* _____

35. The American Academy of Pediatric Dentistry recommends that children have their first dental visit by 1 year of age. *(375)* _____

36. What are the causes of bottle-mouth caries? *(376-377)*

    _____

    _____

    What is the prevention measure for them? *(376-377)* _____

    _____

37. Administration of _____ after age _____ is important to prevent dental caries. *(376)*

38. What is the first-aid measure for traumatic loss of a permanent tooth? *(377-378)*

    _____

    _____

    _____

39. What is the chief difference between the play of several toddlers (ages 1–2 years) and play of several preschoolers (ages 3–5 years)? *(378)*

    _____

    _____

    _____

THINKING CRITICALLY

1. Observe a child in the clinical area. Based on the assessment, determine which of Erikson's stages of development the child is attempting to accomplish. Give at least three examples of observed behavior that support your choice.

2. Using the information provided in Table 15-6 in the textbook and the Food Guide Pyramid (Figure 15-6), develop a meal plan for a 9-year-old child using foods unique to that child's ethnic background.

APPLYING KNOWLEDGE

1. a. Plot the height and weight of the following children on the growth chart (Figure 15-4 in the textbook).

Age	Height	Weight
2 years (boy)	33 in.	26 lbs.
4 years (girl)	38 in.	43 lbs.
8 years (boy)	52 in.	60 lbs.
12 years (girl)	58 in.	65 lbs.

   b. What percentile does each of the above children fall into?
   c. Which child would need further evaluation of his or her growth?

2. Plan a menu for a 4-year-old hospitalized child on a general diet. Include in your plan serving size and how the food is best served.

3. Perform a developmental assessment using the Denver II. Discuss your experience with your classmates.

REVIEW QUESTIONS

1. A child must be able to sit before he can walk. This is an example of which directional pattern of development? *(348)*
    1. Cephalocaudal
    2. Proportional
    3. Proximodistal
    4. Linear

2. One of the most accurate indicators of biologic age is: *(350)*
    1. height.
    2. weight.
    3. bone growth.
    4. teeth eruption.

3. According to Piaget, the 7- to 11-year-old child is at which of the following stages of cognitive development? *(362)*
    1. Sensorimotor
    2. Formal operations
    3. Concrete operations
    4. Proportional

4. The nurse instructs the parent of an infant that dental caries are prevented through the administration of oral: *(376)*
    1. iodine.
    2. fluoride.
    3. sodium.
    4. iron.

Student Name _____

5. Most children are able to feed themselves using a spoon by age: *(372)*
   1. 1 year.
   2. 2 years.
   3. 3 years.
   4. 4 years.

6. The theorist known for his work on moral development is: *(355)*
   1. Freud.
   2. Kohlberg.
   3. Sullivan.
   4. Piaget.

7. A current comic strip depicts a family in which parents, children, and the children's grandfather live together. This is an example of a(n): *(354)*
   1. nuclear family.
   2. alternate family.
   3. extended family.
   4. reconstituted family.

8. Blood cholesterol levels below which level are considered acceptable in children and adolescents? *(370)*
   1. < 170 mg/dl
   2. < 180 mg/dl
   3. < 200 mg/dl
   4. < 220 mg/dl

9. The nurse understands that primary dentition is usually completed by age: *(374)*
   1. 18 months.
   2. 2½ years.
   3. 4 years
   4. 6 years.

10. An infant weighed 7 lbs., 11 oz. at birth. What would the nurse expect this infant to weigh at 12 months of age? *(348)*
    1. 15 lbs.
    2. 20 lbs.
    3. 23 lbs.
    4. 25 lbs.

11. Which of the following statements would have the most positive outcome when the nurse is counseling adolescents on nutrition? *(373)*
    1. "If you don't eat properly now, you may have heart trouble when you get older."
    2. "You will get run down and sick if you don't eat properly."
    3. "Shiny hair and good muscles are linked to good nutrition."
    4. "If you eat nutritiously, you won't have acne."

12. Young children are playing with action figures in the hospital playroom. Closer observation reveals they are playing alongside one another, rather than interacting with each other. The nurse is observing: *(378)*
    1. solitary play.
    2. parallel play.
    3. cooperative play.
    4. creative play.

13. The nurse determines a parent needs additional teaching about nutrition when the parent states: *(376)*
    1. "My 2-year-old child uses a spoon to feed himself."
    2. "I feed my 8-month-old infant iron-fortified cereal."
    3. "My 1-year-old infant falls asleep with a bottle of formula."
    4. "I give my 3-year-old 3 tablespoons of vegetables."

14. The nurse would teach a parent to introduce solid foods to an infant at what age? *(370)*
    1. 3 months.
    2. 6 months.
    3. 8 months.
    4. 10 months.

15. What is the best nursing response to a parent who asks when her 3-month-old infant can switch from iron-fortified formula to milk? *(372)*
    1. "Switch to milk when you introduce solid foods."
    2. "The baby can have milk when she can drink from a cup."
    3. "Milk can be given at 6 months of age."
    4. "Infants can drink milk after their first birthday."

16. A 4-year-old child had a low score on the Denver II. The nurse understands that this finding indicates: *(352)*
    1. the need for further evaluation.
    2. the child has a cognitive impairment.
    3. there is a problem with the child's speech.
    4. the child has a developmental delay.

17. Which statement made by a parent indicates an understanding about a child's dental health? *(377)*
    1. "I give my son a new toothbrush every year on his birthday."
    2. "I rinse the toothbrush bristles in hot water after my son brushes."
    3. "My 1-year-old brushes his teeth all by himself every day."
    4. "I replaced the toothbrush after my son had a sore throat."

18. The nurse is assessing the nutritional status of a 6-year-old child. Which finding suggests the child is well-nourished? *(373)*
    1. Protuberant abdomen
    2. Pale oral mucous membranes
    3. Alert and energetic
    4. Coarse, thin hair

CHAPTER 16

The Infant

Answer Key: Textbook page references are provided as a guide for answering these questions. A complete answer key was provided for your instructor.

LEARNING ACTIVITIES

1. Match the terms in the left column with their definitions on the right (a–h).

_____ Colic *(390)*	a. Closure of the hand when the palm is touched or stroked
_____ Creeping *(388)*	b. Thrusting tongue movements that automatically push food out of the mouth
_____ Extrusion reflex *(392)*	c. Extension of both arms when thrust downward in the prone position
_____ Grasp reflex *(380)*	d. Ability to grasp objects between all fingers of one hand and the opposing thumb of the same hand
_____ Object permanence *(397)*	e. Self-propelled forward movement carrying trunk above and parallel to floor
_____ Parachute reflex *(380)*	f. Accurate and coordinated opposition of index finger and thumb of same hand
_____ Pincer grasp *(380)*	g. Infant can remember that an object exists even if it is out of sight
_____ Prehension *(380)*	h. Unexplained episodes of crying and irritability in an otherwise healthy infant

2. How does sucking benefit a young infant? *(381)*

   a. _____

   b. _____

3. How can the nurse help meet the infant's sucking needs during the following? *(381)*

   a. Oral feedings _____

   _____

   _____

b.   Intravenous fluid therapy _____

_____

_____

4.   a.   The primary goal for normal personality development during infancy is to acquire a sense of _____. *(381)*

b.   What can the nurse teach parents about meeting this need of their infant? *(381)*

_____

_____

5.   Appropriate sensory stimulation is needed to promote what type of infant development? *(381)*

a.   _____

b.   _____

6.   State the approximate age when the following events in an infant's growth and development are likely to occur. *(384-389)*

a.   _____ months: briefly holds head erect and in the midline of body

b.   _____ months: feeds self finger foods

c.   _____ months: should have first DTP (diphtheria, tetanus, pertussis) immunization

d.   _____ months: two lower central incisors; begins to crawl; transfers objects from one hand to the other

e.   _____ months: birth weight tripled; may walk

f.   _____ months: sits alone; pincer grasp

g.   _____ months: walks holding furniture; deliberately throws objects on floor

h.   _____ months: turns from back to side

i.   _____ months: can place a toy in small container

j.   _____ months: "jumps" when in lap of caregiver

7.   a.   Why should most infants not be placed in the prone position for sleep? *(390)*

_____

_____

b.   Give examples of measures to reduce an infant's risk of suffocation. *(390)*

_____

_____

Student Name _____

8. What are three points that the nurse should emphasize to the parents to promote childhood immunization? *(392)*

   a. _____

   b. _____

   c. _____

9. What guidance can the nurse give new parents who are concerned about whether their baby is receiving an adequate diet of breast milk or formula? *(392)*

   a. _____

   b. _____

   c. _____

10. List four assessments that the health care provider may use to gauge the adequacy of an infant's nutrition. *(392)*

    a. _____

    b. _____

    c. _____

    d. _____

11. List health benefits for breastfeeding an infant. *(392)*

    a. _____

    b. _____

    c. _____

    d. _____

12. What food should be avoided until the child is 2 years old? Why should this food be avoided? Explain how you would avoid the food. *(395)*

    _____

    _____

    _____

13. a. What is the current recommendation about when solid foods may be introduced to the infant's diet? *(394)*

    _____

    _____

    b. Why is this a good age to begin introducing solid foods? *(394)*

    _____

    _____

14. a. What is the first solid food usually introduced to the infant? *(394)* _____

    _____

    b. Why is this food good as an introductory solid food? *(394)* _____

    _____

15. How should parents introduce new solid foods so that an infant's tolerance or intolerance of the food can be identified? *(394)*

    _____

    _____

16. List six foods that are usually delayed until the baby is 1 year old. Why is addition of these foods often delayed? *(394)*

    a. _____

    b. _____

    c. _____

    d. _____

    e. _____

    f. _____

17. The United States is becoming more obese, causing multiple health problems in the population. Is feeding an infant a low-fat diet one answer to the problem? Give a reason for your answer. *(395)*

    _____

    _____

THINKING CRITICALLY

1. A mother is concerned because her 4-month-old baby does not seem to be developing as quickly as her sister's baby, who is about the same age. What should the nurse tell this mother about infant development?

CASE STUDIES

1. You are answering questions from the parents of Sarah, a healthy newborn, in each of the following areas. Formulate appropriate parent teaching.
   a. Immunizations (first year) (In addition to your text, see the American Academy of Pediatrics at www.aap.org or the Centers for Disease Control at www.cdc.org for the latest updates about immunization recommendations.)
   b. Sleeping all night
   c. Colic

Student Name_____

2. Danny, 6 months old, is visiting the clinic for his immunizations and checkup. His parents will begin feeding "solid" foods now. What should you teach his parents in each of the following areas?
   a. Order of introducing solid foods
   b. Foods to avoid and how long to avoid them
   c. Avoiding infections acquired from foods

APPLYING KNOWLEDGE

1. Determine the most common infant formulas recommended by physicians or pediatric nurse-practitioners in your clinical facility. What special infant formulas are readily available in the newborn nursery or the pediatric unit and when are these prescribed? Check a grocery, drug, or discount store to compare prices for each formula.

2. Ask a mother who has breastfed a previous child about her experience. Did she pump breast milk and was the milk fed to the baby by bottle? How old was the child when he or she stopped nursing? If the woman you talk with has just given birth to her second or later baby, how does she feel her experience of breastfeeding an older child will affect nursing her newest infant?

3. When caring for an infant in the pediatric unit, talk with parents about their baby's personality. Is their infant irritable, crying with handling or other stimulation, or calm when handled or meeting new people? How does the infant's behavior affect the parents or other family members? What, if any, different infant behavior do they notice while the baby is in the pediatric unit?

4. Ask several parents how they cared for their colicky infant. How long did the infant have colic? How did it affect the family? Was this their first or a later infant?

REVIEW QUESTIONS

1. The priority need in personality development during the first year is to acquire: *(381)*
   1. fear when meeting strangers.
   2. mastering self-feeding.
   3. trust in the primary caregivers.
   4. regular sleeping, waking, and feeding.

2. The primary use of growth and development guidelines is to: *(380-383, 390)*
   1. help parents anticipate their child's changing needs.
   2. compare children of similar ages with each other.
   3. predict general intelligence and school performance.
   4. identify the child who may be mentally retarded.

3. Which developmental milestone is expected for the child's age? *(385, 389)*
   1. Passes a toy from one hand to the other at 3 months.
   2. Uses the root reflex to seek the nipple at 5 months.
   3. Sits steadily and without support at 6 months.
   4. Pulls self to standing position at 10 months.

4. The mother of a 2-month-old is bringing her to the office for a routine checkup and immunizations. She says the baby cries quite a bit but she just lets her cry so she won't become "spoiled." As a nurse, the best response is to: *(384, 390)*
    1. tell the mother she should also lower the lights and play soft music or other "white noise."
    2. explain that babies this young cannot be spoiled, then give her some ideas to help soothe the baby.
    3. encourage the mother to continue helping her baby become more independent.
    4. reassure the mother that she has an irritable baby, but that this phase will not continue for long.

5. The best position for a newborn to sleep is: *(384, 390)*
    1. on the abdomen.
    2. in an infant seat.
    3. with the caregiver.
    4. on the back or side.

6. If a parent wants to microwave formula before feeding, the nurse should: *(393)*
    1. explain that microwaving overheats formula because of higher fat content and can cause severe burns.
    2. tell the parent that cold formula preserves the nutrients better than heating it.
    3. advise the parent to wait until the infant takes at least 8 ounces of formula at each feeding.
    4. teach guidelines for microwaving and caution the parent to test the temperature of the formula before feeding.

7. The primary focus of regular infant health care is to: *(390-393)*
    1. prevent disease.
    2. accelerate development.
    3. delay onset of allergies.
    4. assess growth rate.

8. A mother wants to know if she can keep leftover baby food in a jar. Choose the best nursing response. *(395-396)*
    1. "If you heard a definite 'pop' when opening the jar, refrigerating leftovers is safe."
    2. "Refrigerate the leftover food within 2 hours after it is opened."
    3. "When the baby has eaten all she wants from the jar, promptly refrigerate the remainder."
    4. "Remove the amount of food you think the baby will eat from the jar and refrigerate the rest."

9. A formula often prescribed for the infant who cannot tolerate cow's milk formulas is based on: *(393)*
    1. goat's milk.
    2. soy.
    3. rice.
    4. artificial protein.

10. A nurse counsels a mother who is starting her baby on solid foods that she should wait _____ days before introducing the next food. *(393)*
    1. 1–2
    2. 3
    3. 4–7
    4. 14

Student Name_____

11. Social development that is common for the 2-month-old infant is: *(384)*
    1. responsive smiling.
    2. laughing aloud.
    3. recognizing his/her own name.
    4. anxiety around strangers.

12. When bringing her 9-month-old baby in for a checkup, a new mother asks if she can feed the baby puréed fish since this is a low-fat food that is a staple in the family's diet. The best response of the nurse is: *(394)*
    1. "It is never too early to begin a heart-healthy diet."
    2. "Fish protein is one of the best quality proteins available."
    3. "You can try, but many infants dislike the taste of fish."
    4. "Fish is more likely than other meats to cause allergies."

13. The parents should make safety preparations prior to the time their infant crawls, usually about age: *(387)*
    1. 4 months.
    2. 7 months.
    3. 9 months.
    4. 12 months.

14. Which is the most important teaching about use of the microwave for heating infant food? *(394, 396)*
    1. Use less time than would be needed for larger pieces of food.
    2. Rotate the food two or more times while warming it.
    3. Avoid heating foods that are higher in fat, such as meat.
    4. Test the temperature of any warmed food on the inner wrist.

15. A fruit that should be delayed until after the infant's first birthday is: *(394)*
    1. strawberries.
    2. applesauce.
    3. apricots.
    4. pears.

16. Considering safety when choosing toys for a 5-month-old, one should assume that all of them will go into the baby's: *(386)*
    1. tub.
    2. food.
    3. mouth.
    4. bed.

17. Minor head lag when pulling a 1-month-old infant to the sitting position: *(384)*
    1. is an expected finding.
    2. demonstrates prematurity.
    3. identifies poor nutrition.
    4. suggests developmental delay.

18. A mother is concerned because her 1-year-old, who was 7 pounds (3178 g) at birth is "getting fat." The baby now weighs 21 pounds and all developmental milestones have been reached at appropriate ages. What should the nurse tell the mother about her baby's weight? *(386, 389, 397)*
    1. The weight at 12 months is about twice the birth weight.
    2. The baby's weight gain is what is expected at this age.
    3. A low-fat diet helps avoid being overweight later in life.
    4. Infants normally weigh about 25 pounds by 1 year.

19. The nurse can reassure parents that their infant's colic will probably not last beyond the age of: *(384)*
    1. 1 month.
    2. 3 months.
    3. 6 months.
    4. 9 months.

20. The baby can usually be offered finger foods such as toast or Zwieback crackers beginning at about age: *(387)*
    1. 3 months.
    2. 5 months.
    3. 7 months.
    4. 9 months.

21. A good initial method to deal with a 9-month-old infant who is attracted to a dangerous situation is to: *(388)*
    1. shout a quick, loud "no."
    2. take his favorite toys away.
    3. spank him with one light blow.
    4. distract him from the situation.

CHAPTER 17

The Toddler

Answer Key: Textbook page references are provided as a guide for answering these questions. A complete answer key was provided for your instructor.

LEARNING ACTIVITIES

1. Match the terms in the left column with their definitions on the right (a–g).

   _____ Autonomy *(403)*
   _____ Cooperative play *(411)*
   _____ Egocentric *(410-411)*
   _____ Negativism *(399)*
   _____ Parallel play *(411)*
   _____ Ritualism *(399)*
   _____ Separation anxiety *(401)*

   a. Independent play in company of other children
   b. Playing with other children
   c. Consistent, recurring pattern of behavior
   d. Independent functioning
   e. Thinking in reference to oneself
   f. Frequent reaction of "no"
   g. Protest, despair, and detachment related to temporary absence of caregiver

2. What age is the toddler is expected to achieve each developmental milestone? *(400)*

   a. Can undress self, throws ball _____

   b. All deciduous teeth are erupted; complete bowel and bladder control _____

   c. Imitates adults' activities, holds spoon _____

3. According to Erickson, the major developmental task for the toddler is to acquire _____ and overcome _____ and _____. *(399)*

4. What are the expected average vital signs for a 2-year-old? *(400)*

   a. Pulse: _____ to _____ bpm

   b. Respirations: _____ to _____ breaths/minute

   c. Blood pressure: _____ mm Hg

5. Describe each of these normal developmental processes. How can danger to a child occur related to expected development? Describe observations you have made of children related to each. *(401)*

    a. Separation anxiety

    _____

    _____

    _____

    b. Object permanence

    _____

    _____

    _____

6. What is a good guideline to teach parents about using "time out" with children? *(403)*

    _____

7. List two self-consoling behaviors that toddlers exhibit. *(403)*

    a. _____

    b. _____

8. How should an adult talk to a toddler? Why? *(405)*

    _____

9. List four indications of readiness for toilet training (in any order). *(405)*

    a. _____

    b. _____

    c. _____

    d. _____

10. Bladder training is more likely to succeed if the toddler stays dry for about _____ hours. *(405)*

11. Why is it important to teach the toddler generally recognized words to signal a need to use the bathroom? *(406)*

    _____

    _____

    _____

    _____

Student Name _____

12. a.   What deficiency is more likely to occur if a toddler has excessive milk and too few solid foods? *(406)*

      _____

   b.   This can result in what condition? *(406)* _____

      _____

13. Describe two characteristics of the toddler's eating habits.

   a.   Appetite *(406)* _____

   b.   Food preferences *(406)*_____

14. What guideline can the nurse give parents about serving size of solid foods? *(406)*

   _____

15. List interventions that can assist parents with the toddler who resists bedtime. *(404, Table 17-4)*

   a.   _____

   b.   _____

   c.   _____

   d.   _____

   e.   _____

   f.   _____

16. _____ are the leading cause of childhood death. *(408)*

17. List two methods that are mandated by law to prevent injuries in children. *(408)*

   a.   _____

   b.   _____

CASE STUDY

1.   Tommy is a 2-year-old whose mother is frustrated because of his temper tantrums when he is disciplined. What can you teach Tommy's mother about discipline at his age? How can knowledge of normal growth and development be used to teach his mother about setting limits?

APPLYING KNOWLEDGE

1.   How can you help parents deal with the fears of their toddler? Why is it important for adults to control their own fears around a toddler? If you must do an unfamiliar procedure as a student (such as giving an injection) to a toddler, how do you control your own fears?

2.   How can you use assessment of expected growth and development during the toddler years or other periods of childhood to provide better care when the child is hospitalized?

3. How can parents' knowledge of a child's expected growth and development help protect the child from injury? Give examples of advice you might give to parents of an 18-month-old child, a 24-month-old child, and a 36-month-old child.

4. How does full myelination of the spinal cord relate to success of toilet training?

5. Use growth charts to determine if the physical growth of children you care for in clinical experience is normal.

6. Discuss day care with classmates who are parents. Are they satisfied with the care their children receive? What, if any, problems have they had with day care? What alternatives to day care of young children do classmates use?

REVIEW QUESTIONS

1. A first-time mother is concerned because she believes her 18-month-old son is not growing properly. Assessment indicates that the little boy's height and weight are average for his age. How can the nurse best advise her? *(399-400)*
   1. "He will soon resume the rapid growth of the first year."
   2. "It is normal for a child's growth to slow down after the first year."
   3. "Toddlers grow at inconsistent rates, much like adolescents."
   4. "The physician will do testing if your son's growth remains slow."

2. When helping a toddler choose clothing for the day, the best approach is to: *(399)*
   1. ask him what he wants to wear.
   2. ask which of two appropriate outfits he prefers.
   3. select the best outfit for the weather.
   4. remove all inappropriate clothing from his closet.

3. The position that best facilitates adult-child conversation is: *(405)*
   1. at the child's eye level.
   2. above the child's eye level.
   3. standing while the child sits.
   4. both seated at a small table.

4. When teaching parents of the toddler about eating, the nurse should stress that the toddler: *(406-407)*
   1. prefers a variety of foods mixed on the plate.
   2. must usually be coaxed to eat adequately.
   3. eats one food for a while, then rejects it.
   4. usually enjoys regular addition of new foods.

5. The mother of a 2-year-old asks the nurse whether she should begin toilet training now. The most appropriate nursing response is: *(405-406)*
   1. "Waiting about 6 months will improve the child's success with training."
   2. "Does your child ever wake up dry in the morning?"
   3. "Is it important to you and your family that the child be trained now?"
   4. "It is probably easy to toilet train your child if he will sit on the potty chair."

Student Name_____

6. Automobile child restraint devices should be used when the child: *(408)*
    1. begins sitting in the rear seat.
    2. crawls about in the car.
    3. resists activity restraints.
    4. travels anywhere in the car.

7. Select the toy that is most likely to injure a toddler. *(408-409)*
    1. Balloon
    2. Blocks
    3. Sand box
    4. Pull toy

8. Which is the best description of a 2-year-old's speech and language ability? *(401-402)*
    1. Naming objects precedes the ability to describe what they do.
    2. Some words such as swearing are used because they shock adults.
    3. Talking to the child delays clear speech by limiting time to practice.
    4. The child understands more than he or she is able to verbalize.

9. Choose the best description of physical changes during the toddler years. *(400)*
    1. Head growth slows and chest growth continues.
    2. Muscle size and strength remain steady.
    3. Body temperature regulation is erratic.
    4. Fighting infections is less than during infancy.

10. The nurse can help reduce accidental injuries to toddlers by: *(408)*
    1. providing toys that help accelerate motor development.
    2. teaching parents about expected behavioral changes.
    3. providing written information about common child hazards.
    4. using restraints whenever the child is uncooperative.

11. Select the assessment that should make a parent or health care provider suspect a communication disorder. *(402-403)*
    1. An 18-month-old child does not respond when his name is called.
    2. A 15-month-old child can point to one picture when the parent calls its name.
    3. A 3-year-old child can use plurals and pronouns correctly.
    4. A 16-month-old child cannot use two-word phrases when appropriate.

12. When assessing a 2-year-old child hospitalized for minor day surgery, the nurse should expect that the pulse rate will be about _____ bpm. *(400)*
    1. 60–80
    2. 70-110
    3. 125–135
    4. 120–140

13. When buying shoes for their toddler, parents should choose those that provide: *(405)*
    1. a firm, straight sole to facilitate walking.
    2. a strong arch to prevent "fallen" arches.
    3. protection from objects that might injure the feet.
    4. adequate movement of the heel within the shoe.

14. Choose the recommendation that best helps to promote safety for the toddler. *(410)*
    1. Keep medicines on a shelf rather than on the countertop.
    2. Provide stickers for each phone with the poison control center number.
    3. Advise parents to have a cell phone with them when driving.
    4. Do not use a hair dryer to dry the child's hair after shampooing.

15. A mother asks you what she should do about her 2-year-old child's temper tantrums. The best response is: *(403-404)*
    1. "He is trying to tell you that he needs more attention from you and other important adults."
    2. "If you let him get away with temper tantrums now, he will have more problems later."
    3. "Have you tried rewarding his good behavior?"
    4. "Try putting him in his room for about 30 minutes."

CHAPTER 18

The Preschool Child

Answer Key: Textbook page references are provided as a guide for answering these questions. A complete answer key was provided for your instructor.

LEARNING ACTIVITIES

1. Match the terms in the left column with their definitions on the right (a–f).

   _____ Animism *(415)*

   _____ Artificialism *(415)*

   _____ Centering *(415)*

   _____ Egocentrism *(415)*

   _____ Enuresis *(422)*

   a. Concentrating on a single aspect of an object
   b. Attributing lifelike qualities to inanimate objects
   c. Involuntary urination after the age at which bladder control should have been established
   d. Viewing everything in reference to oneself
   e. Belief that everything is created by people

2. State the following typical vital signs in the preschool child. *(414)*

   a. Pulse: _____ to _____ bpm

   b. Respirations: _____ breaths/minute

   c. Blood pressure: _____ systolic and _____ diastolic

3. According to Piaget, preschool-age children are in the _____ phase of cognitive development. *(414)*

4. List four characteristics of preoperational thinking. *(415)*

   a. _____

   b. _____

   c. _____

   d. _____

5. In the preschool period, the number of words in a child's sentences should equal _____
   _____. *(415)*

6. Masturbation in the preschool child is considered _____. *(418)*

7. Describe the following general characteristics of the 3-year-old child. *(418)*

    a. Sentences are _____ than at age 2 and they can express _____ and ask _____.

    b. They engage in both _____ and _____ play.

    c. May have a _____ attachment to the parent of the opposite sex.

8. A fear that is unique to this age group is a fear of _____. *(419)*

9. Describe the following general characteristics of the 4-year-old child. *(419)*

    a. Can use _____ with success.

    b. Prefers _____ toys.

    c. Plays with friends of the _____ sex.

10. The 4-year-old child is _____ and likes to _____. *(419)*

11. Describe the following general characteristics of the 5-year-old child. *(419-420)*

    a. At age 5, children are more _____ and have more _____.

    b. Height increases by _____ inches and weight increases by _____ pounds.

    c. May begin losing _____ teeth.

    d. Can play games that have _____.

12. Describe three ways children benefit from having limits set on their behavior. *(420)*

    a. _____

    b. _____

    c. _____

13. Effective discipline is designed to shift responsibility for control from the _____ to the _____. *(420)*

14. List three discipline methods that are often effective for the preschool child. *(420-421)*

    a. _____

    _____

    b. _____

    _____

    c. _____

    _____

15. A time-out for a 3-year-old child should last _____ minutes. *(420)*

16. Thumb-sucking will not have a detrimental effect on a child's teeth if the habit is discontinued before _____. *(422)*

Student Name _____

17. Describe the two types of enuresis. *(422)*

    a. Primary _____

    b. Secondary _____

18. List five possible causes of enuresis. *(422)*

    a. _____

    b. _____

    c. _____

    d. _____

    e. _____

19. The _____ age rather than the _____ age of the child should be considered when selecting toys for the child. *(425)*

20. What purpose can an imaginary friend serve for a preschool-age child? *(425)*

    _____

21. Hospitalization can be frightening to the preschool child because they are _____. Their thinking is _____. *(426)*

22. Preschool children cannot fully understand cause and effect and they may perceive illness and hospitalization as _____ for past behavior. *(426)*

Answer as either true (T) or false (F).

23. Hospitalized preschoolers may feel abandoned by their parents. *(426)* _____

24. It would be unusual for a preschooler to have enuresis during a hospitalization. *(426)* _____

25. Having the same nurses care for a hospitalized preschooler will lessen the stress of the experience for the child. *(426)* _____

THINKING CRITICALLY

1. What are appropriate ways to encourage preschool children's desires to do things for themselves while they are hospitalized in your clinical facility?

2. How would you help parents who are concerned because their preschool child uses bad language?

CASE STUDY

1. Sharon Giles is being discharged from the birth center with her second baby. Her 3-year-old son Shawn has visited with her and the baby for several hours since the baby's birth. Sharon expresses concern about Shawn's relationship with the new baby since he has previously been the only child in the home. What guidance should the nurse give Sharon about minimizing Shawn's jealousy during the first few weeks after she and the baby go home?

APPLYING KNOWLEDGE

1. As you care for children in the clinical area, identify examples of egocentrism, animism, and artificialism in their behavior.

2. Does your clinical facility have classes for siblings when a new baby is expected? What is included in the classes?

3. What kinds of nursery schools are available in your area? Are there publicly supported nursery schools for children who are from low-income families?

4. When you care for hospitalized children, are you able to use role modeling to teach parents? If you have not used role modeling, think of appropriate ways to use this parent teaching technique.

5. If your clinical facility has a play therapist, observe this staff member's work with children.

REVIEW QUESTIONS

1. A preschool child falls off the swing and cries, "Bad swing! You made me fall!" This child's response is an example of: *(415)*
   1. egocentrism.
   2. intuition.
   3. animism.
   4. symbolism.

2. Choose the best example of egocentric thinking. *(415)*
   1. "The airplane takes me to Grandma's."
   2. "Water is blue because someone colored it."
   3. "This big box is a truck."
   4. "The moon sleeps during the daytime."

3. The nurse would explain to parents that fears of preschool children are usually: *(419)*
   1. similar to those of older children.
   2. a result of the child's easy distraction.
   3. less intense than when they were younger.
   4. greater than those they had as toddlers.

4. When planning to read with a 5-year-old child, the nurse understands that favorite stories of preschool children are those that relate to their: *(419)*
   1. aggressive tendencies.
   2. self-centeredness.
   3. daily experiences.
   4. relationships with others.

5. A healthy preschool girl asks her parents if she will die. The best response is to tell her that: *(419)*
   1. people do not usually die until they are old.
   2. she does not need to worry about dying.
   3. parents usually die before their children.
   4. she will not die for a long time.

Student Name_____

6. What is the most appropriate advice for the nurse to offer parents who are concerned about their preschooler's masturbation? *(418)*
   1. Remove the child's hands from the genitals.
   2. Try to interest the child in another activity.
   3. Tell the child not to touch himself there.
   4. Ask the child why he is rubbing that area.

7. One effective method of discipline for a preschool child is to: *(421)*
   1. reward the child for good behavior.
   2. give the child a light spanking.
   3. review the reasons for discipline.
   4. stop interacting with the child.

8. Choose the most effective way for parents to deal with a preschool child's jealousy of her new brother. *(421)*
   1. Help her choose toys to share with the new baby.
   2. Remind her of things she can do that the baby cannot.
   3. Explain that she will soon love her new brother.
   4. Ask her to share her room with the new baby at first.

9. A child who sucks his thumb is unlikely to have damage to the mouth if the thumb sucking stops before: *(422)*
   1. 3 years of age.
   2. speech is established.
   3. the first teeth erupt.
   4. the permanent teeth erupt.

10. Choose the most appropriate teaching for parents of a child with enuresis. *(422)*
    1. Enuresis is suggestive of emotional instability in a child.
    2. The child's fluid intake should be restricted during the day.
    3. The child should empty his bladder before going to bed.
    4. A relapse during treatment for enuresis is uncommon.

11. According to Erikson, the developmental task of the preschool period is to achieve a sense of: *(416)*
    1. trust.
    2. autonomy.
    3. initiative.
    4. industry.

12. Which of the following is the best choice for a play activity for a 4-year-old child? *(419)*
    1. Watch a videotape
    2. Play a computer game
    3. Ride a bicycle
    4. Build with blocks

13. Choose the approximate age when children begin playing games that have simple rules. *(420)*
    1. 3 years
    2. 4 years
    3. 5 years
    4. 6 years

14. Bedtime for the preschool child should include: *(418)*
    1. flexibility in the time the child goes to bed.
    2. a period of exercise after dinner.
    3. warm milk.
    4. a quiet activity such as a story.

15. A major cause of health problems in preschool children is: *(423)*
    1. immunization reactions.
    2. communicable diseases.
    3. environmental allergies.
    4. accidental injuries.

CHAPTER 19

The School-Age Child

Answer Key: Textbook page references are provided as a guide for answering these questions. A complete answer key was provided for your instructor.

LEARNING ACTIVITIES

1. Match the terms in the left column with their definitions on the right (a–d).

   _____ Concrete operations *(429)*
   _____ Androgynous *(431)*
   _____ Latchkey child *(434)*
   _____ Preadolescent *(436)*

   a. Period immediately preceding adolescence
   b. Sex role concept that incorporates both masculine and feminine qualities
   c. Logical thinking and an understanding of cause and effect
   d. Unsupervised children left at home after school

2. The school-age child differs from the preschool child in that he or she is more interested in _____ than in fantasy. *(429)*

3. According to Erikson, the school-age period is referred to as the stage of _____. *(429)*

4. Concrete operations involve _____ thinking and an understanding of _____. *(429)*

5. School-age children prefer friends of the _____ sex. *(429)*

6. Give approximate vital sign ranges for the school-age child. *(430)*

   a. Average weight gain: _____ pounds per year

   b. Average increase in height: _____ inches per year

   c. Pulse: _____ to _____ bpm

   d. Respiratory rate: _____ to _____ breaths/minute

   e. Systolic blood pressure: _____ to _____ mm Hg

   f. Diastolic blood pressure: _____ to _____ mm Hg

7. How would the nurse advise parents to answer the school-age child's questions about sex? *(431)*

   _____

   _____

8. Describe information school-age children need in preparation for puberty. *(431)*

   a. Boys _____

   _____

   b. Girls _____

   _____

Answer as either true (T) or false (F).

9. Belonging to a group is important to school-age children. *(433)* _____

10. Latchkey children are at higher risk for accidents. *(434)* _____

11. Describe the following typical characteristics of a 6-year-old child. *(434-435)*

    a. The attention span is _____.

    b. Loss of _____ teeth occurs, along with eruption
       of _____.

    c. Greater exposure to _____ occurs with entry
       into school.

    d. Requires _____ hours of sleep per night.

12. The 7-year-old child prefers toys that are _____
    _____. *(435)*

13. Describe the following typical characteristics of an 8-year-old child. *(435-436)*

    a. Prefers friends of the _____.

    b. Enjoys _____ sports, but is a
       _____.

    c. Secret clubs have strict _____.

14. Describe the following typical characteristics of a 9-year-old child. *(436)*

    a. _____ and _____
       _____ are common behaviors.

    b. _____ sports are popular.

    c. Needs _____ hours of sleep per night.

15. Describe the following typical characteristics of a 10-year-old preadolescent. *(437-437)*

    a. Strives for _____, but will take
       suggestions.

    b. Ideas of the _____ are more important than
       those of the individual.

    c. Takes greater interest in his or her _____.

Student Name_____

16. Describe the following typical characteristics of 11- and 12-year-old preadolescents. *(437)*

    a. This period is one of complete _____.

    b. The child has less ability to _____.

    c. The child has _____ permanent teeth.

17. How would the nurse advise parents of a school-age child about homework? *(440)*

    _____

Answer as either true (T) or false (F).

18. Children with an allergy to animal dander should not have a pet. *(441)* _____

19. Children older than 7 years can be responsible for caring for a pet. *(441)* _____

20. Having a pet can foster a sense of responsibility and encourage socialization for a shy child. *(441)* _____

THINKING CRITICALLY

1. For each category listed below, describe one or two ways the nurse can incorporate the needs of the school-age child into care during hospitalization.
    a. Encouraging decision-making
    b. Need for inclusion in a group

CASE STUDIES

1. Rebecca, 6 years old, is receiving her booster immunizations before starting school. Her mother tells you that she is concerned about how Rebecca will adjust to school because it is the first time she will be away from home for a significant part of the day. How can you help her mother prepare Rebecca for school?

2. Kyle, 10 years old, is hospitalized in skeletal traction with a badly fractured wrist and humerus that he suffered when playing street hockey with his friends. Kyle says he is really unhappy about being away from his friends during summer vacation. The boys spend most of the warm hours of the day at the public pool and either skate or ride their bikes until dark. What safety teaching does Kyle need? How can you use knowledge of preadolescent growth and development to teach Kyle and his family about safety? What can you do to meet his needs for companionship with his friends?

APPLYING KNOWLEDGE

1. Observe how experienced nurses prepare children of different ages for medical procedures. Identify ways they use knowledge of growth and development when caring for children of different ages but with similar medical conditions.

2. Watch television programs and evaluate them critically for positive and potentially harmful influences on children. Consider the following factors:
    a. Stimulating the child's imagination
    b. Materialistic focus
    c. Stereotypes (gender, age, race, and family structure)
    d. Violent content

REVIEW QUESTIONS

1. The school-age child who has few experiences of success is likely to develop a sense of: *(429)*
    1. dependence.
    2. inferiority.
    3. trust.
    4. industry.

2. Which best describes physical growth of the school-age child? *(430)*
    1. Rapid growth occurs from 6–9 years of age and then slows.
    2. Slow growth continues until just before puberty.
    3. Height increases faster than weight.
    4. Height and weight remain stable until the onset of puberty.

3. Choose the normal characteristics of vital signs that the nurse should expect when assessing a 9-year-old girl. *(430)*
    1. Blood pressure and pulse are higher than those of boys the same age.
    2. Blood pressure, pulse, and respirations are close to adult levels.
    3. Blood pressure is higher, but pulse and respirations are lower than the adult.
    4. Blood pressure, pulse, and respirations are higher than those of a 6-year-old girl.

4. How would the nurse advise parents regarding a school-age child's questions about sex? *(431)*
    1. Initiate discussions before the child asks any questions.
    2. Answer questions at the child's level of understanding.
    3. Assure parents the topic will be part of the school curriculum.
    4. Select terms that are used by school-age children.

5. The most significant physical development at age 6 years is: *(434)*
    1. loss of the primary teeth.
    2. elongation of the face.
    3. better infection resistance.
    4. rapid growth in height.

6. Worries and minor compulsions are more common at the age of: *(436)*
    1. 6 years.
    2. 7 years.
    3. 9 years.
    4. 11 years.

7. A preadolescent is more likely to accept her parents' decision if: *(437)*
    1. she understands why her parents made the decision.
    2. the parents do not change decisions once they are made.
    3. the parents carefully control the child's friends.
    4. her friends have values similar to her own family's.

8. Which statement made by a 10-year-old child indicates the need for teaching about living a healthy lifestyle? *(439)*
    1. "I go to the dentist twice a year."
    2. "I wear a helmet when I ride my bike."
    3. "I watch 4 hours of television after school."
    4. "I go to bed at 9:00 PM and get up at 7:00 AM."

Student Name_____

9. The preadolescent girl should have supplies for menstruation: *(431)*
   1. before her first menstrual period.
   2. as soon as she knows how heavy her flow is.
   3. when her friends are prepared for theirs.
   4. about six months after breast development begins.

10. Which characteristic is typical of many 9-year-old children? *(436)*
    1. Enjoy secret codes and rituals with friends.
    2. Start projects, but rarely complete them.
    3. Participate in intense teasing of the opposite sex.
    4. Argue and are bossy toward other children.

11. A group of 8- and 9-year-old boys has formed a "club." The boys have a secret password and handshake before they meet. Parents should interpret this behavior as: *(436)*
    1. typical for children in this age group.
    2. a way to avoid being around adults.
    3. preceding criminal-type gang membership.
    4. rebellion against bossy older children.

12. A father is concerned because his 9-year-old son has developed the habit of wrinkling his nose unconsciously. The nurse should tell the father that his son: *(436)*
    1. may have a nerve problem and should be seen by a physician.
    2. cannot get adequate adult attention without taking this action.
    3. is probably doing this because of unresolved tension.
    4. should be corrected any time he is caught doing this action.

13. A school-age child has an adult "hero" of the same sex. What is the most appropriate interpretation of this behavior? *(435, 439)*
    1. The child feels insecure and inadequate around other children.
    2. Identifying with adults of the same sex is common at this time.
    3. Molestation or sexual abuse by the adult should be considered.
    4. The child is exploring various career and lifestyle options.

14. Which statement characterizes the 8-year-old child? *(436)*
    1. Eight-year-olds are totally disorganized.
    2. They are beginning to take an increased interest in their appearance.
    3. At this age, children are quieter and more modest than the year before.
    4. They like competitive sports, but are poor losers.

CHAPTER 20

The Adolescent

Answer Key: Textbook page references are provided as a guide for answering these questions. A complete answer key was provided for your instructor.

LEARNING ACTIVITIES

1. Match the terms in the left column with their definitions on the right (a–g).

   _____ Adolescence *(444)*
   _____ Androgens *(445)*
   _____ Estrogens *(445)*
   _____ Menarche *(447)*
   _____ Puberty *(447)*
   _____ Growth spurt *(445)*
   _____ Self-concept *(449)*

   a. One's view of oneself
   b. Rapid period of growth in which the body reaches adult height and weight
   c. First menstrual period
   d. Period during which reproductive organs become functional
   e. Female sex hormones
   f. Male sex hormones
   g. Period beginning with appearance of secondary sex characteristics and ending with physical and emotional maturity

2. List the four major tasks of adolescence: *(444)*

   a. _____

   b. _____

   c. _____

   d. _____

3. In the formal operations stage of cognitive development, late adolescents are capable of _____ reasoning. *(444)*

4. One of the strongest needs of adolescents is _____. *(445)*

5. Define *preadolescence*. *(445)* _____

   _____

6. Puberty occurs earlier in which gender? _____ *(445)*

7. The first change of puberty in a boy is _____ _____. *(447)*

8. Boys begin sperm production at about _____ years of age. *(447)*

9. Two important cancer detection tests that are appropriately taught during adolescence are the _____ and _____ self-examinations. *(447)*

10. A girl's first menstrual period is called _____. *(447)*

11. Erikson identifies the major task of adolescence as _____. *(449)*

12. Describe several possible adult outcomes if the adolescent does not achieve his or her own identity. *(449)*

    _____

    _____

    _____

    _____

Answer as either true (T) or false (F).

13. Adolescents think everyone is looking at them. *(451)* _____

14. An adolescent's preoccupation with his or her appearance is a normal behavior. *(451)* _____

15. How can cliques facilitate adolescent peer relationships? *(452)* _____

    _____

16. State ways parents can help their teenager develop increased responsibility in each of the following areas. *(453)*

    a. Routine tasks _____

       _____

       _____

    b. Managing money _____

       _____

       _____

Answer as either true (T) or false (F).

17. Daydreaming is a warning sign of a mental health problem. *(453)* _____

18. An adolescent's cultural background can influence dating behavior. *(454)* _____

19. Sexual curiosity and masturbation are common among adolescents. *(454)* _____

Student Name_____

20. Parents should answer an adolescent's questions about sex truthfully. *(454)* _____

21. Sexual experimentation with same-sex partners during adolescence is a predictor of homosexuality. *(455)* _____

22. List two factors that increase the risk for nutritional deficiencies during adolescence. *(457)*

 a. _____

 _____

 b. _____

 _____

23. An adolescent's diet is most likely to be deficient in which three nutrients? *(457)*

 a. _____

 b. _____

 c. _____

24. An adolescent who follows a vegan diet should be advised to include foods that provide sufficient quantities of which nutrients? *(457)*

 a. _____

 b. _____

 c. _____

 d. _____

 e. _____

 f. _____

25. The primary safety risk to the adolescent is related to use of a(n)_____. *(458)*

26. High school students who participate in competitive sports should have a _____ screening. *(459)*

27. A change in school performance, appearance, and behavior can be a warning sign of _____ _____. *(459)*

THINKING CRITICALLY

1. A 15-year-old girl is at the pediatrician's office for a well-child examination. After you measure her weight, she tells you she is worried about being fat. Her weight is at the 75th percentile for her age. How would you respond to the girl's comment?

2. You are assigned to care for a 14-year-old boy. He responds to your questions with one-word answers. What strategies would you use to establish a rapport with this adolescent?

CASE STUDIES

1. John's mother is worried about the change for the worse in the behavior of her only child. "Our family has always enjoyed many activities together, but now John only wants to be with his friends. He doesn't seem to care that his clothes look bizarre, and yet he's constantly fussing with his hair. He never seems to pay attention. I'm afraid his grades will fall and he won't get into a good college." What advice can you offer John's mother to help her understand her son's behavior?

2. Mary Lou, 15 years old, confides to you that she and her boyfriend have had sex a few times. Mary Lou is concerned about getting pregnant, but does not know much about contraception. She says that talking to her parents about sex and contraception is out of the question. How can you help Mary Lou make responsible decisions concerning her sexuality? What problems have you seen in adolescents who become parents?

APPLYING KNOWLEDGE

1. Observe a group of young adolescents. Identify behaviors in the group that demonstrate the following:
   a. Efforts to develop an identity
   b. Preoccupation with self
   c. Cultural variations

2. Obtain statistics for your state and city about the number of vehicle accidents in which teenagers were involved. If possible, determine how long the young drivers had been licensed.

3. Visit community groups that focus on reducing gang violence among teenagers. Determine the approximate ages of gang members and how they identify themselves to one another and to rival gangs.

4. Obtain local statistics for violent deaths among teenagers. How many of these are thought to be related to gangs?

REVIEW QUESTIONS

1. Younger adolescents often have an awkward appearance because: *(445)*
   1. maturation occurs earlier than in previous generations.
   2. body parts grow and mature at different rates.
   3. growth and development slows during adolescence.
   4. self-consciousness causes the adolescent to slump.

2. A person who does not establish an identity during adolescence is more likely to: *(449)*
   1. conform to a peer group for a prolonged time.
   2. seek close relationships with others.
   3. become insensitive to the needs of others.
   4. have an overly superior self-image.

3. A parent can best help an adolescent make a wise decision by: *(456)*
   1. explaining what he or she would have done when he or she was a teenager.
   2. reviewing problems with the decision after the teenager makes it.
   3. serving as a role model by making the decision for the teenager.
   4. respecting the teenager's decision, even if he or she makes a mistake.

Student Name_____

4. Younger adolescents tend to be egocentric because they are: *(451)*
    1. certain that their parents are ignorant.
    2. believe no-one is paying attention to them.
    3. preoccupied with their physical development.
    4. proud of their greater responsibilities.

5. The adolescent's peer group helps him or her move away from: *(452)*
    1. same sex friendships.
    2. values of his or her family.
    3. individual responsibility.
    4. dependence on his or her family.

6. What is the best nursing response to a parent who is concerned about her 15-year-old's frequent daydreaming? *(453)*
    1. "Daydreaming is a normal adolescent occurrence."
    2. "This behavior is an indicator of adolescent insecurity."
    3. "Your concern is valid because this is a sign of depression."
    4. "It is a way for teenagers to ignore their parents."

7. An adolescent who adopts a strict vegetarian diet is at risk for a deficiency of which nutrient? *(457)*
    1. Carbohydrates
    2. Vitamin C
    3. Protein
    4. Fiber

8. Most accidents in adolescents occur when they: *(458)*
    1. participate in contact sports.
    2. handle guns or knives.
    3. drive a car or other vehicle.
    4. work at part-time jobs.

9. The nurse assessing an adolescent's physical development knows that the Tanner stages describe the: *(449)*
    1. sequence of physical maturation in the adolescent.
    2. change from concrete thinking to abstract thinking.
    3. hormonal changes that cause ovulation and menstruation.
    4. development of a mature gender identity.

10. The major psychosocial task of adolescence is to develop a sense of: *(449)*
    1. sexual orientation.
    2. concern for other people.
    3. family unity.
    4. identity as an individual.

11. A parent is worried because her 14-year-old son seems to be constantly in the bathroom, shampooing and styling his hair. She worries that her son may be homosexual because he is so concerned about his appearance. What is the most appropriate nursing response to the mother's concern? *(455)*
    1. "Homosexual thoughts and experimentation are normal during the early teens."
    2. "Boys are usually more concerned about their athletic abilities than their appearance."
    3. "You should be more concerned about why he does not want to be with his friends."
    4. "Teens are preoccupied with their appearance because of dramatic body changes."

12. What is the best information for the nurse to include in a class for adolescents about healthy eating habits? *(457)*
    1. How to choose foods from the basic food pyramid.
    2. The need to eat three balanced meals per day.
    3. The importance of an adequate diet to better health during adulthood.
    4. Nutrients that are often lacking in an adolescent's diet.

13. What is the best food choice for an adolescent who just finished playing a game of field hockey? *(457)*
    1. Cheeseburger
    2. Chocolate bar
    3. Garden salad
    4. Toasted bagel

CHAPTER 21

The Child's Experience of Hospitalization

Answer Key: Textbook page references are provided as a guide for answering these questions. A complete answer key was provided for your instructor.

LEARNING ACTIVITIES

1. Match the terms in the left column with their definitions on the right (a–d).

   _____ Clinical pathway *(473)*

   _____ Emancipated minor *(478)*

   _____ Regression *(468)*

   _____ Respite care *(478)*

   a. Trained workers come to the home to relieve parents

   b. Loss of an achieved level of functioning to a past level of behavior

   c. Interdisciplinary plan of care that displays progress of the treatment plan for a patient

   d. Adolescent younger than 18 years of age who is no longer under the parents' authority

2. List three advantages of outpatient surgery for the pediatric patient. *(463)*

   a. _____

   b. _____

   c. _____

3. What strategies would the nurse use to prepare a 3-year-old for a procedure? *(464)*

   _____

   _____

   _____

4. A child's reaction to hospitalization depends on: *(465)*

   a. _____

   b. _____

   c. _____

   d. _____

   e. _____

   f. _____

Answer as either true (T) or false (F).

5. Every child reacts differently to the hospital experience. *(465)* _____

6. During hospitalization, a caring and compassionate nurse can take the place of a child's primary caregivers. *(465)* _____

7. Hospitalization can be a positive experience for children. *(465)* _____

8. The three major stressors for children of all ages during hospitalization are: *(465)*

    a. _____

    b. _____

    c. _____

9. Separation anxiety is most pronounced in the _____ stage. *(465)*

10. Match the stage of separation anxiety with the behavior that corresponds with the stage.

    _____ Protest *(465)*
    _____ Despair *(465)*
    _____ Denial *(465)*

    a. Child is sad and depressed.
    b. Child becomes interested in his or her surroundings.
    c. Child cries continuously for "mommy."

11. Assessment of pain is recorded when _____. *(466)*

12. List three nonpharmacologic methods of pain reduction. *(467)*

    a. _____

    b. _____

    c. _____

13. Administration of acetaminophen in quantities exceeding the recommended maximum daily dose can cause damage to the _____. *(467)*

Answer as either true (T) or false (F).

14. Infants and children respond to drugs differently than adults. *(467)* _____

15. Addiction occurs quickly in children receiving opioids for severe pain. *(467)* _____

16. Children 7 years of age and older can be taught to use patient-controlled analgesia. *(467)* _____

17. Administering analgesics on an as-needed schedule is the most effective way to relieve a child's pain. *(467)* _____

18. The nurse must calculate all medication dosages to determine if they are safe to administer to the child. *(467)* _____

Student Name_____

19. Define *conscious sedation.* *(467)* _____

_____

20. What advice would the nurse give to a parent who is concerned that her hospitalized toddler was drinking from a cup and now only wants his bottle? *(468)*

_____

_____

21. List three things the nurse can do to lessen anxiety for the parents of a hospitalized child. *(469-471)*

a.   _____

_____

b.   _____

_____

c.   _____

_____

22. List two ways the nurse can decrease siblings' anxiety when a brother or sister is hospitalized. *(471)*

a.   _____

_____

b.   _____

_____

23. List five topics that are included in a developmental history. *(472)*

a.   _____

b.   _____

c.   _____

d.   _____

e.   _____

24. Give two methods of decreasing the stress of hospitalization for an infant. *(473, 474)*

a.   _____

b.   _____

25. List three examples of transitional objects that can be brought to the hospital for a 15-month-old child. *(474)*

    a. _____

    b. _____

    c. _____

26. What guidelines should the nurse follow for providing explanations about hospital experiences to young children? *(475)*

    a. _____

    b. _____

    c. _____

27. Preschoolers are particularly fearful of _____. *(476)*

28. Explain how the nurse would prepare a preschool child for abdominal surgery. *(476)*

    _____

29. List two ways the nurse can foster a sense of independence for the hospitalized school-age child. *(476)*

    a. _____

    b. _____

30. Following treatments, what should the nurse encourage the school-age child to do? *(477)*

    _____

31. Illness in the young adolescent is seen mainly as a threat to _____ _____. *(477)*

32. What factors should the nurse take into consideration when assigning rooms or roommates for a hospitalized adolescent? *(477)*

    _____

33. Preparation for discharge begins _____. *(478)*

34. What should be included in the documentation when a child is discharged from the hospital? *(478)*

    a. _____

    b. _____

    c. _____

    d. _____

    e. _____

Student Name_____

35. List four suggestions the nurse can give parents who are concerned about behavioral problems arising with their children after hospitalization. *(478)*

   a. _____

   _____

   b. _____

   _____

   c. _____

   _____

   d. _____

   _____

THINKING CRITICALLY

1. Prepare a care plan for a hospitalized toddler. Address the psychosocial needs of the child and parents. Include nursing diagnoses, goals, and interventions.

2. Do you think parents have the right to know if their children are being treated for a sexually transmitted disease? Discuss this with your classmates.

CASE STUDY

1. Scott, 15 months old, is admitted to the hospital with a diagnosis of croup. Both of his parents work and care for two older siblings.
   a. What factors will affect Scott's reaction to hospitalization?
   b. What information will you collect in a developmental history?
   c. How will you use this information to provide nursing care to this toddler?
   d. Scott's mother confides to the nurse that she feels that this hospitalization could have been avoided if she would have taken Scott to the doctor sooner. How can you best answer the mother?
   e. Following admission to the pediatric unit, Scott's parents leave to make arrangements for their other children. Scott cries continuously for his mother. What is your interpretation of this behavior?
   f. Scott's parents take turns spending the night with Scott but are unable to be with him during the day. What fears and behaviors might the parents show because of their separation from Scott?
   g. Scott's 5-year-old sister asks you if her little brother is going to die like when her grandfather was in the hospital. How should you respond to this question?

APPLYING KNOWLEDGE

1. Involve a school-age child in a board game. How effective was this strategy with establishing rapport and communication with the child?

2. While you are in the clinical area, assess a toddler who is alone for signs of separation anxiety. What stage of separation anxiety corresponds to the child's behaviors?

3. Take a hospitalized child to the playroom. Compare the child's behavior while in the playroom to behavior in the hospital room.

4. Discuss with your peers how you feel when parents do not come to visit their hospitalized child. What could be some reasons for their not visiting?

5. Determine the laws in your state governing the treatment of minors.

REVIEW QUESTIONS

1. Separation anxiety is most pronounced in which age group? *(465)*
   1 Infants
   2. Toddlers
   3. Preschool children
   4. Adolescents

2. The mother of a hospitalized toddler could best explain when she will return by saying, "I will be back: *(466)*
   1. in 3 hours."
   2. after your nap."
   3. before six o'clock."
   4. before you know it."

3. In most instances, unpleasant treatments on children should take place in the: *(464-465)*
   1. playroom.
   2. emergency room.
   3. patient's room.
   4. treatment room.

4. A 2-year-old who is anxious about hospitalization will probably benefit most from which intervention? *(474)*
   1. A visit from Bozo the clown
   2. Having her favorite toy brought from home
   3. Having her favorite foods served at lunch
   4. Opening a new gift each day

5. Which child is most likely to feel their illness is punishment for something they have done wrong? *(476)*
   1. Toddler
   2. Preschool
   3. School-age
   4. Adolescent

6. Which intervention is most appropriate to reduce a young child's anxiety related to upcoming surgery? *(471)*
   1. Do not tell the child that he or she is having surgery.
   2. Arrange for the child to meet the surgeon.
   3. Schedule a visit of the surgical area preoperatively.
   4. Give the child a ride on the stretcher before surgery.

Student Name_____

7. Parental consent for minors is not always necessary for treatment in which situation? *(478)*
    1. Minor cuts and abrasions
    2. Psychologic disorders
    3. Communicable diseases
    4. Sexually transmitted diseases

8. The mother of a 3-year-old child is concerned because he has returned to diapers since he has been hospitalized although he had been potty trained. What is the best nursing response to the mother? *(468)*
    1. "This is very unusual and I'm sure it is temporary."
    2. "Keep him in his training pants and don't give in to him."
    3. "Regression is normal in a sick child."
    4. "Perhaps he has some type of urinary infection."

9. The nurse's best approach to prepare a toddler for a painful procedure is to: *(464, 474)*
    1. be truthful if it will be painful.
    2. avoid frightening him by not telling him it might hurt.
    3. begin preparing early so that he can ask questions.
    4. have his mother explain what will happen.

10. What action would the nurse take when a hospitalized school-age child begins to act out? *(476)*
    1. Place the child in a private room.
    2. Discipline the child by having restrictions put in place.
    3. Provide positive direction and consistency.
    4. Ignore the behavior because this is an expected reaction.

11. After performing a painful procedure on an infant, the nurse should: *(464)*
    1. swaddle the infant.
    2. feed the infant.
    3. return the infant to the parent.
    4. change the infant's diaper.

12. The nurse would expect a common reaction to hospitalization for a 4-year-old child to be: *(476)*
    1. anger.
    2. depression.
    3. guilt.
    4. fear.

13. The nurse understands that a hospitalized school-age child should be allowed to participate in his or her own care in order to: *(476)*
    1. decrease fear of bodily injury.
    2. increase self-esteem.
    3. allow some control.
    4. increase responsibility.

14. Because of distance, the family of a young child cannot be at the hospital with her. What is the most appropriate advice for the nurse to offer the family? *(474)*
    1. Hire a private duty nurse to stay with the child.
    2. Bring in family photographs and special toys.
    3. Do not tell the child that they will not be visiting.
    4. Do not call the child because it would be upsetting.

15. What is the best nursing approach to decrease a preschooler's anxiety about having his blood pressure measured? *(464)*
    1. Take the blood pressure while the child is sleeping.
    2. Ask the child's mother to take the blood pressure.
    3. Demonstrate the procedure on a doll prior to performing it on the child.
    4. Tell the child that big boys and girls do not cry when they have their blood pressure taken.

16. A child is receiving morphine sulfate for pain management. What is the most appropriate response to parents who are concerned their child will become addicted to the medication? *(467)*
    1. "Addiction to narcotics is rare in children."
    2. "Is there a family history of drug addiction?"
    3. "The dosage is insufficient to produce addiction."
    4. "This is the best medication to control your child's pain."

17. An 18-month-old child has been crying for "Mommy" since the parent left several hours ago. How would the nurse interpret the toddler's behavior? *(465)*
    1. This is the child's first separation from his mother.
    2. The child is experiencing separation anxiety.
    3. The illness is causing the child to have severe pain.
    4. The child is detached from his father.

Student Name _____

CHAPTER 22

Health Care Adaptations for the Child and Family

Answer Key: Textbook page references are provided as a guide for answering these questions. A complete answer key was provided for your instructor.

LEARNING ACTIVITIES

1. Match the terms in the left column with their definitions on the right (a–d).

   _____ Broviac catheter *(504)*
   _____ Heparin lock *(504)*
   _____ Parenteral fluids *(505)*
   _____ TPN *(505)*

   a. A device to keep a vein open for intermittent medication administration
   b. Given by a route other than the digestive tract
   c. Hyperalimentation
   d. Tiny, flexible tube inserted into a vein in the chest for long-term intravenous administration

2. What is implied when a parent or guardian gives his or her written informed consent for a child to receive medical treatment? *(481)*

   _____

3. A consent form must be signed by the _____, the _____, and a _____. *(481)*

4. The nurse acts as a _____ in ensuring proper consent has been signed _____ a procedure and that the child is given an age-appropriate explanation of the procedure. *(481)*

5. List six safety measures applicable to the hospitalized child. *(482)*

   a. _____

   _____

   b. _____

   _____

   c. _____

   _____

d. _____

_____

e. _____

_____

f. _____

_____

6. Name four safety hazards to avoid when caring for a hospitalized child. *(483)*

a. _____

_____

b. _____

_____

c. _____

_____

d. _____

_____

7. Identify three factors the nurse must consider when selecting the method for transporting a child from the pediatric unit to the radiology department. *(483)*

a. _____

b. _____

c. _____

8. Name two procedures for which the nurse might use a mummy restraint for an infant. *(483)*

a. _____

b. _____

9. What is the purpose of the personal history survey? *(484)*

_____

_____

Answer as either true (T) or false (F).

10. Bradycardia is often the first sign of shock in infants and children. *(484)* _____

11. Hypotension is an early sign of shock in children. *(484)* _____

12. Bradycardia is considered a medical emergency in infants and young children. *(485)* _____

13. Medication dosages in children are determined by the child's weight. *(485)* _____

Student Name_____

14. A _____ fontanel may indicate dehydration and a _____ fontanel may indicate increased intracranial pressure. *(485)*

15. Apical pulses are advised for children under age _____ years and should be counted for _____ seconds. *(486)*

16. The width of the blood pressure cuff should cover _____ of the upper arm. *(486)*

17. Fever is defined as a temperature over _____°F/_____°C. *(489)*

18. Why is it important to obtain an accurate weight measurement for infants and young children? *(485)*

_____

_____

19. To accurately measure the temperature of a 4-year-old child using a tympanic thermometer, the nurse would gently pull the pinna _____. *(490)*

20. Describe the procedure for weighing an infant. *(492)*

_____

_____

_____

_____

21. Describe the procedure for collecting a urine specimen from an infant. *(492)*

_____

_____

_____

_____

_____

22. What is the purpose of a lumbar puncture? *(494)*

_____

_____

23. Explain how a nurse should position a child for a lumbar puncture. *(494)*

_____

_____

_____

_____

_____

24. What information should be recorded after a lumbar puncture? *(495)*

_____

_____

_____

25. _____ is the most important variable in predicting response to any drug therapy. *(495)*

26. Why are drugs metabolized more slowly by infants and young children? *(495)*

_____

27. Use the formula for dimensional analysis to calculate the following medication dosage: A physician ordered amoxicillin 0.25 grams. The pharmacy provides a bottle labeled amoxicillin 500 mg per 5 ml.

    How much medication would the nurse administer? *(498)* _____

28. Determine if the dosage in question #27 is safe for a young child who weighs 33 pounds. The *PDR* states 14-18 mg/kg/dose is a safe dose for young children. *(498)* _____

29. Describe the procedure for administering medication to an infant with an oral syringe. *(500)*

_____

_____

_____

30. Compare the procedure for administering ear drops to children under 3 years of age and children 3 years of age and older. *(501)*

_____

_____

_____

_____

_____

31. Which site would the nurse use to administer an intramuscular injection to an infant? *(502)*

_____

    Why is this the preferred site? _____

_____

32. The maximum volume that can be injected in one site to infants is _____. *(503)*

33. _____, _____, and
    _____ catheters are tiny, flexible rubber tubes inserted into a vein in the chest to establish long-term intravenous therapy. *(504)*

Student Name_____

34. How frequently does the nurse assess a child's intravenous infusion? *(505)* _____

35. Total parenteral nutrition is given to children who: *(505)* _____

_____.

36. What is the appropriate nursing action when the nurse observes brown fluid draining from an infant's gastrostomy tube? *(506)*

_____

_____

_____

37. Describe the procedure for suctioning a child with a tracheostomy. *(510)*

_____

_____

_____

_____

_____

_____

_____

_____

38. List five signs that might indicate a problem in a tracheostomy patient. *(510)*

a. _____

b. _____

c. _____

d. _____

e. _____

39. What emergency equipment should be kept at the bedside of a tracheotomy patient? *(510)*

_____

_____

40. What information should be included in the documentation when assessing a child with a tracheotomy? *(510)*

a. _____

b. _____

c. _____

d. _____

e. _____

41. What is the Heimlich maneuver? *(515)*

_____

42. How is the Heimlich maneuver performed on an unconscious child who is lying down? *(515)*

_____

43. Prior to surgery, infants should not be maintained on NPO status longer than _____ to _____ hours because of the risk of _____. *(515)*

THINKING CRITICALLY

1. You are assisting a registered nurse who is going to start intravenous fluids on a 3-month-old infant. The mother is crying and is not sure if she wants to be with the infant or to remain outside the room during the procedure. How could you support this mother?

APPLYING KNOWLEDGE

1. Where would the following items and areas be found in the clinical setting?
   a. blood pressure machine
   b. diapers
   c. emergency cart
   d. intake and output sheet
   e. IV soluset
   f. oral medication syringe
   g. playroom
   h. procedure manual
   i. scales
   j. thermometer
   k. treatment room
   l. urine collection bag

2. Assist a registered nurse when she starts an IV on a child.

3. Care for a child with a tracheotomy tube.

4. Care for a child receiving gastrostomy tube feedings.

5. Care for a child with an IV infusing.

REVIEW QUESTIONS

1. The nurse is aware of which variation in pulse and respiration rates of children as compared to adults? *(486)*
   1. Lower than adults
   2. Same rates as adults
   3. Higher than adults
   4. Lower at birth, but higher by age 3 years

Student Name _____

2. What is the best choice for the nurse to mix with an unpleasant-tasting medication? *(498)*
   1. Orange juice
   2. Milk
   3. Jelly
   4. Cereal

3. An infant's diaper weighs 30 g. How many milliliters would the nurse record on the intake and output sheet? *(507)*
   1. 15
   2. 30
   3. 60
   4. 45

4. When caring for a tracheotomy patient, the nurse would: *(510)*
   1. limit suctioning to no more than 15 seconds.
   2. apply suction as the catheter is being inserted.
   3. use a suction catheter that is approximately the same diameter as the tracheotomy tube.
   4. replace the suction catheter and water used to clear the catheter at the end of the shift.

5. A child weighing 35.5 pounds has a medication order for phenytoin PO at 8:00 AM. The recommended pediatric dosage is 3–5 mg/kg/day. A safe dosage for this child would be: *(498)*
   1. 75 mg.
   2. 105 mg.
   3. 150 mg.
   4. 200 mg.

6. What is the best way for the nurse to weigh an infant? *(492)*
   1. Completely naked
   2. Wearing a dry diaper
   3. Wrapped in a receiving blanket
   4. Lightly dressed

7. The neonate exposed to prolonged high oxygen concentrations is at risk for damage to which part of the body? *(513)*
   1. Heart
   2. Eyes
   3. Brain
   4. Kidneys

8. The nurse assessing a child's vital signs would count both the pulse and respirations for _____ seconds. *(486)*
   1. 15
   2. 30
   3. 45
   4. 60

9. The nurse planning to measure a child's blood pressure would choose a cuff that covers: *(486)*
   1. one-half of the upper arm.
   2. one-third of the upper arm.
   3. two-thirds of the upper arm.
   4. the entire upper arm.

10. A 4-month-old infant's pulse rate is 140 beats per minute. How would the nurse interpret this assessment finding? *(486)*
    1. Within normal limits
    2. Tachycardia
    3. Bradycardia
    4. Life-threatening situation

11. The preferred intramuscular injection site for infants is the: *(515)*
    1. deltoid.
    2. ventrogluteal.
    3. vastus lateralis.
    4. dorsogluteal.

12. The maximum volume that can be given by intramuscular injection at one site to older infants and small children is: *(502)*
    1. 0.1 ml.
    2. 0.5 ml.
    3. 1.0 ml.
    4. 1.5 ml.

13. An expectant parent tells the nurse, "I am planning to put the baby in an antique crib." What advice on crib safety would the nurse offer to this parent? *(483)*
    1. The crib slats should be no more than 2⅜ inches apart.
    2. Measure the crib slats to be sure they are at least 2⅜ inches wide.
    3. There should be 2⅜ inches between the mattress and the side rail.
    4. Keep the side rails 2⅜ inches higher than the baby's length.

14. After administering a gastrostomy tube feeding, how would the nurse position an infant? *(511)*
    1. Left side
    2. Supine
    3. Right side
    4. Prone

15. The nurse appropriately positions a 7-year-old child for a lumbar puncture: *(494)*
    1. prone with knees flexed to the chest.
    2. laying on the side in a fetal position.
    3. sitting up and hugging the nurse.
    4. supine with the head flexed to the chest.

16. The nurse explained to a parent the procedure for administering an oral antibiotic to an infant. Which statement made by the parent indicates a correct understanding of the information? *(500)*
    1. "I should use a syringe with a short, thin needle."
    2. "Put the medicine in a bottle with a small amount of water."
    3. "Use an oral syringe to place the medicine in the side of the mouth."
    4. "Bring the medicine cup to the baby's lips to drink slowly."

17. What is the most appropriate nursing intervention to prepare a 4-year-old child for placement of an intravenous line? *(508)*
    1. Tell the child that he needs the IV a few hours before the procedure.
    2. Provide an explanation for why he needs to have an IV.
    3. Let the child know that crying is okay when something hurts.
    4. Show the child the mummy restraint that will be used.

CHAPTER 23

The Child with a Sensory or Neurological Condition

Answer Key: Textbook page references are provided as a guide for answering these questions. A complete answer key was provided for your instructor.

LEARNING ACTIVITIES

1. Match the terms in the left column with their definitions on the right (a–j).

_____ Enucleation *(527)*	a. Short period of sleep following a seizure
_____ Hyperopia *(525)*	b. Farsighted
_____ Myringotomy *(522)*	c. Incision of the tympanic membrane
_____ Nystagmus *(532)*	d. Involuntary movement of the eye
_____ Papilledema *(532)*	e. Adduction of arms, flexed on chest with wrists flexed, hands fisted, and lower extremities extended and adducted
_____ Postictal lethargy *(535)*	f. Edema and inflammation of the optic nerve
_____ Strabismus *(526)*	g. Temporary disturbance of the brain followed by a period of unconsciousness
_____ Concussion *(542)*	h. Removal of the eye
_____ Decerebrate *(543)*	i. Rigid extension and pronation of the arms and legs
_____ Decorticate *(543)*	j. Cross-eyed

2. An acute infection of the external ear canal is called _____ or _____. *(520)*

Answer as either true (T) or false (F).

3. When a child has otitis externa, the tympanic membrane is erythematous. *(520)* _____

4. Prolonged exposure to moisture is a precipitating factor of otitis externa. *(520)* _____

5. Otitis media frequently occurs after a child has an upper respiratory infection. *(521)* _____

6. Explain why infants are more prone to ear infections than older children. *(521)*

_____

_____

_____

7. List the main symptoms of otitis media. *(521)*

_____

_____

8. List two possible complications of recurrent episodes of otitis media. *(522)*

    a. _____

    b. _____

9. Describe the treatment of otitis media. *(522)*

_____

_____

10. What teaching should be done when antibiotics are prescribed for children with acute otitis media? *(522)*

_____

_____

_____

11. Complete bilateral deafness is usually discovered during _____, but partial deafness may be unrecognized until _____. *(523)*

12. Identify assessment findings that might indicate a hearing problem. *(523)*

    Infant

    a. _____

    b. _____

    Older Child

    a. _____

    b. _____

13. List three strategies the nurse can use when caring for a hospitalized school-age child who has a hearing impairment. *(523)*

    a. _____

    b. _____

    c. _____

14. Identify one strategy to relieve a child's discomfort resulting from a change in altitude or barometric pressure during airplane descent. *(524)*

_____

_____

Student Name _____

15. During a visual assessment, the nurse should observe the eyes for: *(525)*

    a. _____

    b. _____

16. Visual acuity can be tested by _____ to _____ years of age. *(525)*

17. Explain the goal of treatment of amblyopia. *(525)*

    _____

    _____

    _____

18. Why might a child be embarrassed when being treated for amblyopia? *(525)*

    _____

    _____

    _____

19. Untreated strabismus can result in _____. *(526)*

20. Describe the procedure for wiping secretions from the eye in the child with conjunctivitis. *(526)*

    _____

    _____

21. How would the nurse position a child who has a hyphema? *(527)*

    _____

22. List the clinical manifestations of retinoblastoma. *(527)*

    _____

23. Neural tube development occurs about the _____ to _____ week of fetal life. *(527)*

24. What medication, when used during a viral illness, has been linked to Reye's syndrome? *(527)*

    _____

25. Which two immunizations are recommended to prevent sepsis for all children between 2 months and 4 years of age? *(530)*

    a. _____

    b. _____

26. List five signs and symptoms of meningitis. *(530-531)*

    a. _____

    b. _____

    c. _____

    d. _____

    e. _____

27. Nursing measures for the child with meningitis include: *(531)*

    a. _____

    b. _____

    c. _____

    d. _____

28. List two measures the nurse should take to decrease stimuli when caring for a child with meningitis. *(531)*

    a. _____

    b. _____

29. The majority of brain tumors in children are located in the _____ _____. *(532)*

30. The manifestations of a brain tumor are directly related to the _____ and _____ of the tumor. *(532)*

31. Most brain tumors create increased _____, producing symptoms such as _____, _____, _____, and _____. *(548)*

32. Preoperative care of a child with a brain tumor should address what body image issue? *(532-533)*

    _____

33. Febrile seizures occur in response to a _____. *(533)*

34. What should the nurse observe and record after a seizure? *(533)*

    a. _____

    b. _____

    c. _____

    d. _____

    e. _____

    f. _____

    g. _____

Student Name _____

35. Match each classification of seizure with its description (a–d).

_____ Generalized tonic-clonic seizure *(534)*   a. Temporary loss of awareness
_____ Absence seizure *(534)*   b. Can be manifested by motor activities, sensory
_____ Partial seizure *(534)*   signs, or psychomotor activity
_____ Myoclonic seizure *(534)*   c. Repetitive muscle contractions
                                                      d. Has three phases: aura, seizure, and postictal
                                                         period

36. What is the term meaning a series of convulsions rapidly following one another? *(536)*

   _____

37. The most common cause of status epilepticus is _____. *(536)*

38. List four common causes of cerebral palsy. *(537)*

   a. _____

   b. _____

   c. _____

   d. _____

39. List three clinical manifestations that might indicate a child has cerebral palsy. *(537)*

   a. _____

   b. _____

   c. _____

40. List three precautions that should be taken when the nurse is feeding a toddler with cerebral palsy. *(538)*

   a. _____

   b. _____

   c. _____

41. Nurses can contribute to the prevention of mental retardation by promoting: *(541)*

   a. _____

   b. _____

   c. _____

   d. _____

42. Identify the following illustrations as decorticate posturing or decerebrate posturing. *(542)*

    a. _____

    b. _____

43. The four components of a neurologic check are: *(543)*

    a. _____

    b. _____

    c. _____

    d. _____

44. List three questions you might ask a 4-year-old child to help determine his or her level of consciousness. *(543)*

    a. _____

    b. _____

    c. _____

45. Vital sign changes suggestive of increased intracranial pressure include: *(543)*

    a. _____

    b. _____

    c. _____

46. Priorities for treatment of a child who experienced near-drowning include immediate treatment of _____, _____, and _____. *(546)*

THINKING CRITICALLY

1. You are assigned to care for a 5-year-old child who has a seizure disorder. When you walk into her room, she is watching TV. You are asking the child some questions when her body stiffens. She is unresponsive. Thirty seconds later, her arms and legs begin contracting and relaxing. What type of seizure is this child experiencing? What should you do at this time?

Student Name_____

CASE STUDIES

1. Kevin, age 6 months, is admitted to the hospital with meningitis. He is placed in isolation, an IV is started, and he is on seizure precautions.
   a. How would Kevin be positioned for a lumbar puncture?
   b. What changes in Kevin's spinal fluid would confirm a diagnosis of meningitis?
   c. Kevin's temperature is 102.4° F. For what other signs and symptoms would the nurse assess?
   d. State at least 6 nursing interventions for Kevin.

2. Two-year-old Andrew has chronic otitis media with effusion. Audiometric testing shows a mild hearing loss. He is scheduled for a myringotomy with insertion of tympanoplasty tubes.
   a. How will this surgery improve Andrew's hearing?
   b. What should Andrew's parents know about care of a child with tympanoplasty tubes inserted?

APPLYING KNOWLEDGE

1. While in the clinical area, care for a child who is on seizure precautions. What are some of the special procedures you followed?

2. Assist with vision screening in your local school district.

3. Visit your local Easter Seal Society and observe the therapy of children with cerebral palsy. Find out what resources are available for these children.

REVIEW QUESTIONS

1. What information would the nurse give to parents of a young child following surgical insertion of tympanostomy tubes? *(522)*
   1. Decongestants are needed for several weeks.
   2. Avoid getting water in the child's ears.
   3. Position the child on his back for sleep.
   4. Use cotton swabs to clean the ears.

2. Visual acuity can be checked by age: *(525)*
   1. 2½–3 years.
   2. 3–4 years.
   3. 4–5 years.
   4. 5–6 years.

3. Early signs of Reye's syndrome include: *(529)*
   1. diarrhea and headache.
   2. vomiting and lethargy.
   3. nausea and malaise.
   4. hyperactivity and vomiting.

4. When taking the history of a child with encephalitis, it is important to note recent: *(532)*
   1. cat scratches.
   2. exposure to poison ivy.
   3. respiratory infection.
   4. drug therapy.

5. Cerebral palsy is: *(537)*
    1. a form of mental retardation that does not improve with treatment.
    2. a nonprogressive disorder that affects the motor centers of the brain.
    3. always caused by a birth injury occurring in early gestational births.
    4. related to lack of early childhood stimulation and is irreversible.

6. Which factor is most likely to trigger seizures in a child with epilepsy? *(536)*
    1. High-fat diet
    2. Hypothermia
    3. Sensitivity to light
    4. Loud noises

7. The nurse recognizes which of the following as signs and symptoms of meningitis? *(531)*
    1. Diarrhea and stiff neck
    2. Hyperactivity and vomiting
    3. Irritability and fever
    4. Loss of vision and nausea

8. A 7-month-old child had a febrile seizure. Which statement would the nurse give to the infant's parents? "Febrile seizures: *(533)*
    1. rarely occur before an infant's first birthday."
    2. indicate an underlying neurological problem."
    3. are usually controlled with phenobarbital."
    4. rarely develop into epilepsy."

9. The nurse monitors fluid intake and output in children with a head injury in order to: *(546)*
    1. prevent renal damage.
    2. control cerebral edema.
    3. prevent aspiration.
    4. decrease headaches.

10. Nursing care for a child following a generalized tonic-clonic seizure would include: *(534)*
    1. attempting to hold the tongue.
    2. administering oxygen.
    3. restraining extremities.
    4. turning on his or her side.

11. The nurse teaching parents about adverse effects of Dilantin would explain this medication can cause: *(535)*
    1. drowsiness.
    2. gum overgrowth.
    3. blurred vision.
    4. liver toxicity.

12. Which nursing action is appropriate when caring for a hospitalized child who is hearing-impaired? *(523)*
    1. Speak in a loud, clear tone.
    2. Stand close to the child and speak slowly.
    3. Speak at eye level with the child.
    4. Speak in an exaggerated tone.

13. An infant brought to the emergency room with a high fever, irritability, and a high-pitched cry would immediately be evaluated for: *(531)*
    1. retinoblastoma.
    2. Reye's syndrome.
    3. neuroblastoma.
    4. meningitis.

14. An appropriate nursing intervention for an infant with bacterial meningitis is: *(531)*
    1. restrain the infant when awake.
    2. position the infant on the right side.
    3. keep the room quiet and indirectly lit.
    4. place in isolation until discharged.

15. What is the best action for the nurse to take when a child has a Glasgow coma scale score of 8? *(543)*
    1. Tell the charge nurse immediately.
    2. Change the position of the child.
    3. Chart the results of the assessment.
    4. Stimulate the child.

16. Which question will elicit the best information to determine a plan of care during hospitalization for a 5-year-old child who is mentally retarded? *(541)*
    1. "Can the child dress herself?'
    2. "Is she toilet trained?"
    3. "What is her favorite activity?"
    4. "What is her bedtime routine?"

17. What is the priority for the care of a child with decreased level of consciousness resulting from a head injury? *(547)*
    1. Maintain a patent airway.
    2. Prevent skin breakdown.
    3. Monitor fluid balance.
    4. Perform passive range-of-motion exercises.

18. What is an appropriate nursing intervention for feeding a child with spastic-type cerebral palsy? *(538)*
    1. Touch the tip of the tongue with the spoon.
    2. Stroke downward under the chin area.
    3. Feed with a rubber-coated spoon.
    4. Tilt the head backward 30 degrees.

CROSSWORD PUZZLE

Across

3. Involuntary arching of the back due to muscle contraction *(531)*
6. A short period of sleep following a seizure *(535)*
11. Involuntary, purposeless movements *(538)*
13. A group of nonprogressive disorders that affects the motor centers of the brain *(537)*
14. Inflammation of the brain *(531)*

Down

1. A movement characterized by an alternating contraction and relaxation of muscles *(533)*
2. A reading disability that involves a defect in the cortex of the brain that processes graphic symbols *(525)*
4. Systemic response caused by bacteria in the bloodstream *(530)*
5. Removal of the eye as the standard treatment for retinoblastoma *(527)*
7. A reduction in or loss of vision in a child who strongly favors one eye *(525)*
8. The presence of blood in the anterior chamber of the eye *(527)*
9. Sudden, intermittent episodes of altered consciousness, lasting seconds to minutes *(533)*
10. A condition where there is a lack of coordination between the eye muscles that direct movement of the eye *(526)*
12. A movement characterized by muscle contraction *(533)*

24 The Child with a Musculoskeletal Condition

CHAPTER 24

Answer Key: Textbook page references are provided as a guide for answering these questions. A complete answer key was provided for your instructor.

LEARNING ACTIVITIES

1. Match the terms in the left column with their definitions on the right (a–h).

_____ Genu varum *(550)*	a. Limited neck motion due to shortening of the sternocleidomastoid muscle
_____ Osteomyelitis *(556)*	b. Bow-legged or knees turned outward
_____ Contusion *(551)*	c. Knock-kneed or knees turned inward
_____ Sprain *(551)*	d. Tearing of subcutaneous tissue that results in hemorrhage, edema, and pain
_____ Strain *(551)*	e. A microscopic tear to a muscle or tendon
_____ Genu valgum *(550)*	f. Infection of the bone
_____ Osteosarcoma *(561)*	g. Bone tumor
_____ Torticollis *(563)*	h. Ligament that is torn or stretched away from the bone

2. Assessment of the musculoskeletal system in children who can walk includes: *(550)*

   a. _____

   b. _____

   c. _____

   d. _____

3. It is normal for toddlers to have a _____ gait. *(550)*

4. How would the nurse test the strength of a child's extremities? *(550)*

   _____

Answer as either true (T) or false (F).

5. A newborn's feet may turn inward or outward. *(550)* _____

6. Children who do not walk independently by 12 months of age should be evaluated for a musculoskeletal problem. *(550)* _____

7. Young children may appear "bow-legged" until 5 years of age. *(550)* _____

8. A neurological assessment is part of a comprehensive musculoskeletal assessment. *(550)* _____

9. List three types of traction used for children. *(551)*

    a. _____

    b. _____

    c. _____

10. Identify three differences in the skeletal system of a child as compared to an adult. *(551)*

    a. _____

    b. _____

    c. _____

11. The major signs of a muscle sprain are _____,
    _____, and _____. *(551)*

12. Describe the treatment of a soft tissue injury. *(551-552)*

    _____

    _____

    _____

    _____

13. Match the types of fractures in the left column with their definitions on the right (a–d).

    _____ Simple *(552)*
    _____ Compound *(552)*
    _____ Greenstick *(552)*
    _____ Spiral *(553)*

    a. Bone is broken but the skin over the area is not broken
    b. Caused by forceful twisting motion.
    c. Open fracture in which the wound in the skin leads to the broken bone
    d. Incomplete fracture

14. Bryant's traction is used for treating fractures of the femur in children under _____ years of age or under _____ to _____ pounds. *(553)*

15. You are performing a neurovascular assessment on a young child in Bryant's traction. Name three findings on the neurovascular assessment that should be reported immediately to the nurse in charge. *(554)*

    a. _____

    b. _____

    c. _____

Student Name_____

16. What is Volkmann's ischemia? *(554)*

_____

_____

17. Explain Russell's traction. *(553)*

_____

_____

_____

_____

_____

_____

18. How is nursing care for a child in skeletal traction different from that for a child in skin traction? *(553)*

_____

_____

19. Complete the following traction-related statements. *(553)*

   a.   Weights are hanging _____.

   b.   Weights are out of reach of _____.

   c.   Ropes are on the _____.

   d.   Knots are not resting against _____.

   e.   Bed linens are not on _____.

   f.   _____ is in place.

   g.   Apparatus does not touch the _____ of the _____.

20. A priority nursing responsibility in the care of a child with a cast or in traction is _____
_____. *(555)*

21. A neurovascular assessment of the toes of a child with a fracture who has a cast or Ace bandage includes checking for: *(555)*

   a.   _____

   b.   _____

   c.   _____

   d.   _____

   e.   _____

   f.   _____

22. Pain at the trauma site that is not relieved by analgesics may be a sign of _____ . *(556)*

23. A child is receiving intravenous antibiotics for treatment of osteomyelitis. What is a nursing responsibility related to this treatment? *(560)*

_____

24. The most common type of muscular dystrophy is _____ . *(560)*

25. List three signs that might indicate a child has muscular dystrophy. *(560)*

a. _____

b. _____

c. _____

26. List two clinical manifestations of slipped femoral capital epiphysis. *(560)*

a. _____

b. _____

27. What would the nurse tell the parents about the prognosis of Legg-Calvé-Perthes disease in their child? *(561)*

_____

_____

_____

_____

28. A diagnosis of osteosarcoma is confirmed through a _____ . *(561)*

29. What are the goals of care of juvenile rheumatoid arthritis? *(562)*

a. _____

b. _____

c. _____

d. _____

e. _____

30. The two types of scoliosis are _____ and _____ . *(563)*

31. The Milwaukee brace must be worn _____ hours a day. *(563)*

32. Screening for scoliosis should be done before _____ . *(564)*

Student Name _____

33. What does a screening examination involve? *(564)*

_____

_____

_____

_____

34. A child with scoliosis who needs a spinal fusion has special needs related to immobilization. Identify two nursing interventions to prevent gastrointestinal complications from immobility in the postoperative period. *(564)*

    a. _____

    b. _____

35. A parent asks you for guidelines to help prevent sports injuries in a child who is in competitive sports. List four guidelines. *(565)*

    a. _____

    b. _____

    c. _____

    d. _____

36. What are shin splints? *(565)*

_____

_____

37. When a nurse suspects child abuse, he or she must _____

    _____. *(566)*

38. What guideline for documentation should the nurse follow when caring for a child who has been abused? *(568)*

_____

_____

THINKING CRITICALLY

1. Nurses who care for abused children may have negative feelings toward the adult who abused the child. Examine your thoughts on this issue. Consider how supporting the adult will ultimately help the child.

CASE STUDY

1. Two-year-old Kimberly is admitted to the hospital with a fractured femur. She is placed in Bryant's traction.
   a. Kimberly's mother asks why this particular type of traction is used. How should the nurse reply?
   b. What particular areas of Kimberly's body would be assessed? Provide rationales.
   c. What are some diversional activities the nurse could plan for the child? Base the plan on knowledge of growth and development.

APPLYING KNOWLEDGE

1. While in the clinical area, care for a child in traction.

2. Screen a 10-year-old girl for scoliosis.

3. Label the following bones on Figure 24-1 in the textbook. Check your answers with an anatomy textbook.
   a. femur
   b. tibia
   c. fibula
   d. ulna
   e. radius
   f. coccyx
   g. clavicle
   h. humerus

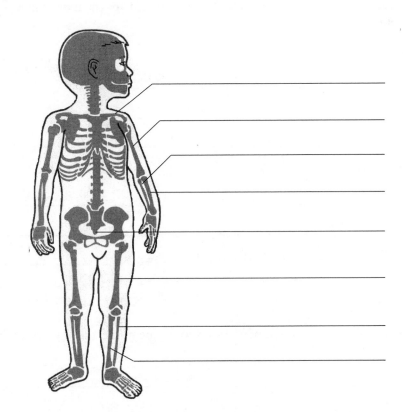

4. Help a child who is immobilized by a musculoskeletal condition plan his diet.

5. Give skin care to a child with skeletal traction.

6. Plan a presentation on sports injury prevention for school-age children with your classmates.

Student Name_____

REVIEW QUESTIONS

1. One of the most common causes of death in a child with muscular dystrophy is: *(560)*
   1. renal failure.
   2. osteomyelitis.
   3. cardiac failure.
   4. liver disease.

2. Which type of traction would the nurse expect to be used for a 20-month-old child who has a fractured femur? *(553)*
   1. Buck extension
   2. Bryant's
   3. Russell's
   4. Ninety-ninety

3. The nurse is aware that a fracture involving the epiphyseal plate in long bone can result in: *(553)*
   1. reduced red blood cell production.
   2. excessive calcium storage.
   3. impaired bone growth.
   4. delayed bone healing.

4. When a child is referred to a physician after scoliosis screening, the plan is to defer treatment and watch the child. The nurse determines that the child's curvature must be less than: *(563)*
   1. 10 degrees.
   2. 20 degrees.
   3. 30 degrees.
   4. 40 degrees.

5. Which is an expected assessment finding in a child with suspected scoliosis? *(564)*
   1. Prominent clavicle
   2. Expiratory wheeze
   3. Asymmetry of the shoulders
   4. Delayed breast development

6. Which disease is usually inherited as an X-linked disorder? *(560)*
   1. Legg-Calvé-Perthes disease
   2. Scoliosis
   3. Juvenile rheumatoid arthritis
   4. Duchenne's muscular dystrophy

7. The nurse is reinforcing the physician's explanation of treatment for Legg-Calvé-Perthes. What information would the nurse review with parents? *(561)*
   1. Buck's extension traction
   2. Muscle strengthening with weights
   3. Surgery to stabilize the joint
   4. Ambulation-abduction casts or braces

8. The nurse completed a neurovascular check on a child in Russell's traction for a fractured femur. Which finding should be reported to the charge nurse? *(554)*
    1. Foot is warm to the touch.
    2. Can wiggle toes.
    3. Toes feel tingly.
    4. Capillary refill of toes < 3 seconds.

9. The treatment of osteomyelitis includes the use of: *(556-557)*
    1. steroids.
    2. antibiotics.
    3. traction.
    4. hydrotherapy.

10. The development of iridocyclitis is a complication of: *(562)*
    1. Legg-Calvé-Perthes disease.
    2. osteomyelitis.
    3. juvenile rheumatoid arthritis.
    4. scoliosis.

11. An appropriate nursing action when caring for a child in Bryant's traction is to: *(552-553)*
    1. remove the weights when bathing.
    2. support the weights when the bed is moved.
    3. position the child so the buttocks touch the bed.
    4. position the child's legs at right angles to the body.

12. Which is a priority nursing diagnosis for an adolescent treated for osteosarcoma? *(561)*
    1. Risk for infection
    2. Posttrauma syndrome
    3. Disturbed body image
    4. Risk for trauma

13. A toddler has been walking independently for one month. Observation of a toddler's gait reveals the child's feet are wide apart and the gait is unsteady. How would the nurse interpret this finding? *(550)*
    1. The child appears to have genu varum.
    2. Orthotic devices in the shoes will improve the gait.
    3. A comprehensive neurological assessment is indicated.
    4. This is a normal gait for a child in the toddler age group.

14. The mother of an infant born with congenital torticollis tells the nurse she is concerned that her child will always have limited neck motion. What is the best nursing response to the mother's concern? *(563)*
    1. "Your child will always need to wear a neck brace."
    2. "Surgery is the treatment of choice to correct the problem".
    3. "The condition will most likely resolve by 2–6 months."
    4. "There is nothing you can do to improve the condition."

15. A child is being removed from the home of an abusive parent. The child is crying and a co-worker wonders if this could be a sign that the child was not abused. The nurse understands that the child: *(568)*
    1. would not be crying if they had been abused in the home.
    2. will mourn the loss of the family, even if there was abuse.
    3. is seeking attention from any available adult.
    4. doesn't really understand what is happening.

Student Name _____

16. Which statements by a mother might indicate future problems related to the care of a newborn infant? *(567)*
    1. "I am happy that my mother will be here for a few weeks. I will have time to recuperate and adjust to my larger family."
    2. "May I call you with questions? This is my first child and although I feel prepared, I am feeling frightened by the responsibility."
    3. "The baby cries all the time. She doesn't seem to like me. I didn't think it would be like this. Sometimes I think she is just trying to irritate me."
    4. "Our baby has colic. We are taking turns rocking her and getting up with her at night. When will we get a full night of sleep?"

17. What would be the priority nursing intervention when a nurse is caring for a child wearing an ace bandage for a sprained ankle? *(552)*
    1. Insure the ankle is elevated on a pillow.
    2. Perform a neurovascular assessment.
    3. Apply a fresh ice pack to the sprained ankle.
    4. Determine when the child received analgesia.

CHAPTER 25

The Child with a Respiratory or Cardiovascular Disorder

Answer Key: Textbook page references are provided as a guide for answering these questions. A complete answer key was provided for your instructor.

LEARNING ACTIVITIES

1. Match the terms in the left column with their definitions on the right (a–f).

   _____ Clubbing *(589)*
   _____ Stridor *(575)*
   _____ Polycythemia *(600)*
   _____ Status asthmaticus *(587)*
   _____ Dysphagia *(574)*
   _____ Shunt *(597)*

   a. Blood flow through an abnormal opening
   b. Harsh, high-pitched sound on inspiration
   c. Asthma attack that is not responsive to drugs
   d. Increased red blood cells
   e. Compensatory response indicating a chronic lack of oxygen
   f. Difficult swallowing

2. The common cold is also known as _____. *(573)*

3. List five measures that can relieve the symptoms of the common cold. *(574)*

   a. _____

   b. _____

   c. _____

   d. _____

   e. _____

4. The child with a strep throat is no longer infectious when _____. *(575)*

5. What is the treatment for sinusitis? *(575)* _____

6. Define the term *croup*. *(575)*

   _____

   _____

   _____

7. Describe the clinical course of laryngotracheobronchitis. *(576)*

_____

_____

_____

_____

_____

8. What advice would you give a parent about home care of a child with croup? *(576)*

_____

_____

_____

_____

_____

9. If epiglottitis is suspected, what nursing responsibility must be instituted? *(576)*

_____

10. The treatment of choice for a child with epiglottitis is a _____ or
    _____. *(576)*

11. List the common signs and symptoms of bronchiolitis. *(577)*

    a. _____

    b. _____

    c. _____

    d. _____

12. What position facilitates breathing for the infant with bronchiolitis? *(577)*

    _____

13. Respiratory syncytial virus (RSV) is spread by _____. *(577)*

14. RSV can survive for more than _____ hours on countertops, tissues, and soap. *(577)*

15. The priority nursing diagnosis for an infant hospitalized with RSV infection is _____
    _____. *(578)*

16. List four of the possible signs of respiratory distress. *(575, 578)*

    a. _____

    b. _____

    c. _____

    d. _____

Student Name_____

17. What are some of the common signs and symptoms of pneumonia? *(579)*

    a. _____

    b. _____

    c. _____

    d. _____

18. Home care for a child with pneumonia involves: *(579)*

    a. _____

    b. _____

    c. _____

19. The removal of the tonsils and adenoids should wait until the child is at least _____ years of age. *(579)*

20. What signs and symptoms are indicative of bleeding in the postoperative tonsillectomy patient? *(581)*

    a. _____

    b. _____

    c. _____

    d. _____

21. What are the characteristic signs of allergic rhinitis? *(582)*

    _____

22. Describe the pathologic changes that take place in asthma. *(582)*

    _____

    _____

    _____

    _____

    _____

23. List five signs and symptoms of an acute asthma episode. *(583)*

    a. _____

    b. _____

    c. _____

    d. _____

    e. _____

24. Name three bronchodilators used in the management of asthma. *(584)*

    a. _____

    b. _____

    c. _____

25. Name three antiinflammatory medications used in the management of asthma. *(584-585)*

    a. _____

    b. _____

    c. _____

26. What would the nurse teach the family of a child with asthma about controlling allergens in the child's bedroom? *(585)*

    _____

    _____

    _____

    _____

27. Why should a child with asthma use a spacer with a metered dose inhaler? *(587)*

    _____

28. Cystic fibrosis is inherited as a _____ trait. That means _____ parent(s) carry the gene for the disease. *(587)*

29. Describe how cystic fibrosis affects the child's respiratory system. *(588, 589)*

    _____

    _____

    _____

    _____

30. Describe the stools of a child with cystic fibrosis. *(588)*

    _____

31. What physiologic changes take place in the pancreas of a child with cystic fibrosis? *(589)*

    _____

    _____

    _____

32. A _____ is the test of choice for diagnosing cystic fibrosis. *(589)*

Student Name_____

33. List three ways respiratory complications can be decreased in patients with cystic fibrosis. *(589-590)*

   a. _____

   _____

   b. _____

   _____

   c. _____

   _____

34. Discharge teaching of a child with cystic fibrosis should include instructions about: *(594)*

   a. _____

   b. _____

   c. _____

   d. _____

   e. _____

   f. _____

35. Children with cystic fibrosis should receive which vitamin supplements? *(594)*

   _____

36. What is the best way to prevent bronchopulmonary dysplasia? *(594)*

   _____

37. The nurse teaches parents to place infants in the _____ position for sleep. This measure reduces the risk of _____. *(595)*

38. List five signs that indicate an infant may have a congenital heart defect. *(596)*

   a. _____

   b. _____

   c. _____

   d. _____

   e. _____

39. _____ are the leading cause of death among the congenital anomalies during the first year of life. *(597)*

40. Heart defects can be classified as lesions that: *(597)*

    a. _____

    b. _____

    c. _____

41. Match the types of heart defects on the left with their definitions on the right (a–d).

    _____ Ventricular septal defect *(599)*   a. Narrowing of the aortic arch or the descending
    _____ Coarctation of the aorta *(599)*   aorta
    _____ Atrial septal defect *(598)*   b. Opening between the right and left ventricles
    _____ Patent ductus arteriosus *(599)*   c. Failure of the ductus arteriosus to close
                                                   d. Opening between left and right atria

42. When a ventricular septal defect is present, increased pressure in the _____ ventricle forces blood back into the _____ ventricle. The defect causes a _____ to _____ shunting of blood. *(599)*

43. Why are prophylactic antibiotics given to children with ventricular septal defects? *(599)*

    _____

44. Describe the characteristic murmur associated with patent ductus arteriosus. *(599)*

    _____

45. What is the classic sign of coarctation of the aorta? *(599)*

    _____

    _____

46. Describe the four defects that make up tetralogy of Fallot. *(600)*

    a. _____

    b. _____

    c. _____

    d. _____

47. Explain why polycythemia develops in children with tetralogy of Fallot. *(600)*

    _____

    _____

48. How would the nurse position an infant experiencing a paroxysmal hypercyanotic episode? *(600)*

    _____

Student Name_____

49. List four signs and symptoms of congestive heart failure. *(602)*

    a. _____

    b. _____

    c. _____

    d. _____

50. Respirations over _____ breaths/minute in a newborn at rest indicate distress. *(602)*

51. Nursing goals when caring for a child with a heart defect include: *(602)*

    a. _____

    b. _____

    c. _____

    d. _____

    e. _____

    f. _____

52. List three nursing actions you could take to conserve the energy of a child with a heart defect. *(602)*

    a. _____

        _____

    b. _____

        _____

    c. _____

        _____

53. Children receiving diuretics must have their serum _____ monitored closely. *(603)*

54. List four foods high in potassium. *(603)*

    a. _____

    b. _____

    c. _____

    d. _____

55. List the signs and symptoms of digitalis toxicity. *(603)*

    a. _____

    b. _____

    c. _____

    d. _____

    e. _____

56. What are the classic symptoms of rheumatic fever? *(603-604)*

    a. _____

    b. _____

    c. _____

    d. _____

57. Rheumatic fever can be avoided by identification of _____ infections and treatment with _____. *(605)*

58. What advice would you give an adolescent who shows a consistently high blood pressure reading? *(606)*

    _____

59. Kawasaki's disease causes _____ of the vessels in the cardiovascular system, which can result in _____. *(606)*

60. Name three medications that may be used in the treatment of Kawasaki's disease. *(607)*

    a. _____

    b. _____

    c. _____

THINKING CRITICALLY

1. You are caring for a 1-month-old infant with a ventricular septal defect who is in congestive heart failure. When you measured the infant's apical heart rate before his 8:00 AM dose of Lanoxin, it was 112 bpm. Should you administer the Lanoxin?

2. Plan for the discharge of a child newly diagnosed with cystic fibrosis. Include diet, medication, respiratory care, and psychologic care of the child and the parents.

3. Develop a teaching plan for 17-year-old adolescent with a serum cholesterol level of 199 mg/dl.

Student Name_____

CASE STUDIES

1. Six-year-old Jasmine is admitted to the hospital with a diagnosis of asthma. She is restless, has difficulty breathing, and is wheezing. She has numerous allergies.
   a. Jasmine relates that she has been taking allergy shots and they have removed many of the objects she is allergic to from their home. Explain each of these methods of allergy treatment.
   b. What position should Jasmine assume to decrease respiratory distress?
   c. The physician wants Jasmine to have increased fluid intake. What liquids should be encouraged and which should be avoided?
   d. Jasmine wants to participate in the swim team at school. What should the nurse tell her about asthma and exercise?
   e. Explain to Jasmine how to use a metered dose inhaler for her medication.

2. Alicia, an 8-year-old child, is admitted to the hospital with cystic fibrosis. She has a history of chronic pulmonary and sinus problems.
   a. Alicia takes an oral pancreatic enzyme. When should she take this medication?
   b. Alicia has extensive lung disease. What measures would improve respiration?
   c. What type of diet would be ordered for Alicia?
   d. Alicia's appetite has markedly decreased. What can be done to increase her intake?

APPLYING KNOWLEDGE

1. Observe a cardiac catheterization in the clinical area.

2. Care for a child with cardiac disease.

3. Care for a child who has had cardiac surgery.

4. Care for a child in an oxygen tent who has a respiratory disease.

5. Care for a child who has had a tonsillectomy.

6. Admit a child to the unit who has asthma.

7. Teach a child with cystic fibrosis about respiratory care and diet.

8. Become certified in pediatric CPR.

9. While in the clinical area, locate the unit's emergency cart and review the contents.

REVIEW QUESTIONS

1. What is the most common congenital heart defect occurring in children? *(599)*
   1. Ventricular septal defect
   2. Coarctation of the aorta
   3. Atrial septal defect
   4. Patent ductus arteriosus

2. What is the best method of feeding an infant in congestive heart failure from a large ventricular septal defect? *(602)*
   1. Space feedings at least every 3–4 hours.
   2. Give frequent, large feedings.
   3. Feed intravenously.
   4. Feed smaller amounts more frequently.

3. If the pulse of a newborn is below _____ bpm, Lanoxin is withheld. *(603)*
    1. 120
    2. 110
    3. 100
    4. 90

4. When an infant is receiving Lanoxin, the nurse would be alert to which finding as a sign of toxicity? *(603)*
    1. Fluid retention
    2. Diarrhea
    3. Nausea and vomiting
    4. Weight loss

5. A nurse's responsibility when a child is receiving diuretics is to: *(603)*
    1. withhold fluids.
    2. monitor serum electrolyte levels.
    3. place on seizure precautions.
    4. check the dosage with another nurse before administering.

6. A child who is hypertensive is identified during routine screening. The nurse would expect which plan of care to be implemented? *(606)*
    1. The child is started on a diuretic.
    2. Beta-adrenergic blockers are prescribed.
    3. An exercise and diet program is developed.
    4. A blood pressure measurement is scheduled in 4 weeks.

7. An infant with tetralogy of Fallot becomes hypercyanotic. The nurse would place the infant in the _____ position. *(600)*
    1. high Fowler's
    2. Trendelenburg
    3. side-lying
    4. knee-chest

8. An appropriate intervention for a child with bronchiolitis is: *(577)*
    1. isolation.
    2. increased fluids.
    3. antihistamines.
    4. increased solids.

9. What is the best liquid for the nurse to give to a child who has had a tonsillectomy? *(581)*
    1. Apple juice
    2. Milk
    3. Pepsi
    4. Lemonade

10. The nurse determines a parent understands diet teaching for a child with cystic fibrosis when she states the child should eat which type of diet? *(594)*
    1. High calorie, high protein
    2. High calorie, low protein
    3. Low calorie, high protein
    4. Low calorie, low protein

Student Name_____

11. The nurse places a child with croup in an environment of high humidity for which effect? *(595)*
    1. Decrease the possibility of dehydration
    2. Decrease risk of spreading the infection
    3. Decrease mucosal swelling
    4. Decrease body temperature

12. An appropriate nursing action when a child is suspected of having epiglottitis is to: *(576)*
    1. avoid examination of the pharynx.
    2. collect a throat culture.
    3. place the child on the right side.
    4. institute isolation precautions.

13. The nurse observes a child who had a tonsillectomy a few hours earlier is swallowing frequently. What is the appropriate action for the nurse to take? *(579, 581)*
    1. Offer the child a drink.
    2. Reposition the child.
    3. Give the child an analgesic.
    4. Notify the physician.

14. Which information would be included in a teaching plan for a child with asthma? *(585)*
    1. Avoid exercise and sports activities.
    2. Keep house humidity above 50%.
    3. Identify early signs of an asthma attack.
    4. Decrease the amount of liquids taken after 6:00 PM.

15. An infant with a congenital heart abnormality would most likely experience: *(596)*
    1. difficulty feeding.
    2. difficulty sleeping.
    3. normal weight gain.
    4. decreased blood pressure.

16. The nurse would expect the parent of an infant with croup to describe the infant's cough as: *(575)*
    1. dry.
    2. barking.
    3. productive.
    4. quiet.

17. Which medication is not useful when a child is experiencing an asthma attack? *(584)*
    1. Albuterol
    2. Cromolyn sodium
    3. Corticosteroids
    4. Theophylline

18. A congenital heart defect that results in decreased pulmonary blood flow is: *(600)*
    1. atrial septal defect.
    2. aortic stenosis.
    3. tetralogy of Fallot.
    4. patent ductus arteriosus.

19. The nurse measuring an infant's blood pressure finds it is higher in the arms than the legs. The finding is associated with which congenital heart defect? *(599)*
    1. Ventricular septal defect
    2. Coarctation of the aorta
    3. Hypoplastic left heart syndrome
    4. Tetralogy of Fallot

CROSSWORD PUZZLE

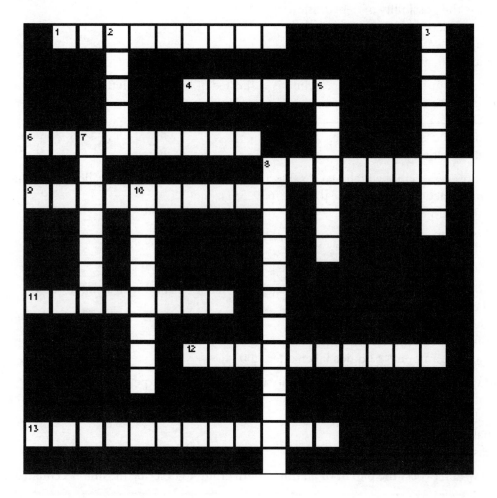

Across

1. Increased respiratory rate *(579)*
4. A cold *(573)*
6. Painful swallowing *(574)*
8. Obstruction to blood flow caused by narrowing of a vessel *(599)*
9. Prevents the alveoli from collapsing during respiration after birth *(572)*
11. Inflammation of the heart *(604)*
12. Increased airway responsiveness in asthma is intermittent or _____ *(582)*
13. Increased number of red blood cells *(600)*

Down

2. General term applied to a number of conditions with symptoms of a brassy cough and varying degrees of stridor *(575)*
3. Compensatory response to chronic lack of oxygen *(589)*
5. Air sacs in the lungs *(578)*
7. Harsh, high-pitched sound heard on inspiration *(575)*
8. Amount of blood ejected during one heart contraction *(602)*
10. Heart disease occurring after birth *(601)*

Student Name _____

CHAPTER 26

The Child with a Condition of the Blood, Blood-Forming Organs, or Lymphatic System

Answer Key: Textbook page references are provided as a guide for answering these questions. A complete answer key was provided for your instructor.

LEARNING ACTIVITIES

1. Match the terms in the left column with their definitions on the right (a–g).

   _____ Alopecia *(621)*   a. Red blood cells (RBCs)
   _____ Erythrocytes *(610)*   b. Pinpoint hemorrhagic spots beneath the skin
   _____ Hemarthrosis *(618)*   c. White blood cells (WBCs)
   _____ Leukocytes *(610)*   d. Platelets
   _____ Petechiae *(611)*   e. Hemorrhage into a joint cavity
   _____ Purpura *(611)*   f. Loss of hair
   _____ Thrombocytes *(611)*   g. Larger hemorrhagic spots in the skin

2. State the functions of the following blood components. *(610-611)*

   a. Leukocytes _____

   b. Erythrocytes _____

   c. Thrombocytes _____

3. List the causes of iron-deficiency anemia. *(612)*

   a. _____

   b. _____

   c. _____

   d. _____

4. List four food sources with high iron content. *(612)*

   a. _____

   b. _____

   c. _____

   d. _____

5. List the major signs and symptoms of iron-deficiency anemia. *(612)*

    a. _____

    b. _____

    c. _____

    d. _____

6. Infants should be screened for iron-deficiency anemia at _____ and _____ months of age. *(612)*

7. What instructions would you give to a parent about administering an iron supplement to a toddler? *(612)*

    _____

    _____

    _____

8. Describe the stools of a young child receiving an iron supplement. *(612)*

    _____

9. What should the nurse tell a parent about formula and milk intake during the first year of life? *(612)*

    _____

    _____

    _____

10. Sickle cell disease is most prevalent in the _____ population. *(614)*

11. List four factors that might trigger a sickle cell crisis. *(614)*

    a. _____

    b. _____

    c. _____

    d. _____

12. Explain the difference between sickle cell trait and sickle cell disease. *(614)*

    _____

    _____

    _____

    _____

Student Name _____

13. The child with sickle cell disease inherits the abnormality from _____
_____. *(614)*

14. List the types of sickle cell crises. *(615)*

   a. _____

   b. _____

   c. _____

   d. _____

15. What is the most common test used to screen for sickle cell disease? *(616)*

   _____

16. Why is meperidine not recommended for children with sickle cell disease? *(616)*

   _____

17. Patient-controlled analgesia can be used for the child over _____ years of age to manage pain caused by sickle cell crisis. *(616)*

18. List two priority goals when caring for a child with sickle cell disease. *(616)*

   a. _____

   b. _____

19. The mainstay of treatment for thalassemia major is _____
_____. *(617)*

20. Children with thalassemia major develop _____ as a result of treatment. *(617)*

21. Hemophilia is inherited as a _____trait. *(618)*

22. Hemophilia A is caused by a deficiency of _____. *(618)*

23. A classic symptom of hemophilia is _____, which is a hemorrhage into a _____. *(618)*

24. The principal therapy for hemophilia is to prevent _____ by replacing the missing factor. *(618)*

25. _____ is a nasal spray that can stop bleeding and may be the treatment of choice for mild cases of hemophilia. *(618)*

26. When bleeding occurs in a child with hemophilia, the traditional approach is to: *(618)*

   a. _____

   b. _____

   c. _____

   d. _____

27. Describe the clinical manifestations of idiopathic thrombocytopenic purpura (ITP). *(619)*

_____

_____

_____

_____

28. The most common form of childhood cancer is _____. *(620)*

29. Leukemia results in the uncontrolled growth of _____

_____. *(620)*

30. Explain the pathologic changes that take place when a child has leukemia. *(620)*

_____

_____

_____

31. List seven of the possible presenting signs and symptoms of leukemia. *(620)*

   a. _____

   b. _____

   c. _____

   d. _____

   e. _____

   f. _____

   g. _____

32. List the five phases of treatment of leukemia. *(621)*

   a. _____

   b. _____

   c. _____

   d. _____

   e. _____

33. List some of the common side effects of chemotherapy. *(621)*

   a. _____

   b. _____

   c. _____

   d. _____

   e. _____

Student Name _____

34. Identify three nursing interventions appropriate for a 10-year-old girl who is worried about alopecia associated with chemotherapy. *(621)*

    a. _____

    b. _____

    c. _____

35. List five signs of a transfusion reaction. *(622)*

    a. _____

    b. _____

    c. _____

    d. _____

    e. _____

36. If a child showed signs of a transfusion reaction, the nurse's initial action would be to _____
    _____. *(622)*

Answer as either true (T) or false (F).

37. Hodgkin's disease is a malignancy of the lymph system. *(622)* _____

38. The presenting sign of Hodgkin's disease is usually pain in the neck and shoulders. *(622)* _____

39. The treatment of Hodgkin's disease involves chemotherapy and radiation therapy. *(623)* _____

40. Following a splenectomy, the child faces the long-term risk of serious _____. *(623)*

41. Describe the preschooler's response to the death of a sibling. *(628)*

    _____

42. The primary fear of dying children younger than 5 years of age is _____
    _____. *(628)*

43. Children develop an understanding of death as permanent around age _____ years. *(628)*

THINKING CRITICALLY

1. Develop a nursing care plan for a child with sickle cell disease experiencing a vaso-occlusive crisis.

2. Review the genetic implications of sickle cell disease by answering the following questions:

   Results of hemoglobin electrophoresis show that an infant has sickle cell anemia. The infant's parents desire to have several more children. When both parents have the sickle cell trait, what are the chances that:
   a. a child will have sickle cell anemia?
   b. a child will carry the sickle cell trait?
   c. a child will have neither the disease nor the trait?
   d. Will the child's gender affect whether the child has the disease? Why or why not?

3. Review the genetic implications of hemophilia when a mother is a carrier of the hemophilia gene and the father does not have the disease.
   a. What are the chances that a son will have the disease?
   b. What are the chances that a daughter will be a carrier?
   c. Why does the child's gender affect whether he or she can manifest this disease?

CASE STUDY

1. Lauren, a 5-year-old girl, is hospitalized with acute lymphocytic leukemia (ALL). She is receiving chemotherapy and has been placed in a private room.
   a. What special precautions should be taken with a child who is immune-suppressed?
   b. Lauren develops ulcerations in her mouth. What can the nurse do to relieve discomfort and promote healing of the oral mucosa?
   c. Lauren is to receive a unit of packed red blood cells. For what signs and symptoms of a reaction should the nurse observe and what action would be taken if a reaction occurred?

APPLYING KNOWLEDGE

1. While in the clinical area, care for a child who has cancer and is receiving chemotherapy.

2. While in the clinical area, care for a child who is experiencing sickle cell crisis.

3. Observe a bone marrow aspiration being performed.

4. Speak with a pediatric nurse who works with children who have cancer about her feelings when a child dies.

5. Visit the Ronald McDonald House in your city. Discuss with your classmates the setting and the services.

6. Discuss with your classmates your feelings when you must cause discomfort to a child in order to help him or her.

7. Develop a family education sheet on preventing iron deficiency anemia.

REVIEW QUESTIONS

1. By what age do children realize that death is final and permanent? *(628)*
   1. 3 years
   2. 5 years
   3. 7 years
   4. 10 years

2. Iron absorption is increased by taking it with: *(612)*
   1. orange juice.
   2. cereal.
   3. milk.
   4. eggs.

Student Name_____

3. It is recommended that iron-fortified formula be given to infants through age: *(618)*
   1. 3 months.
   2. 6 months.
   3. 9 months.
   4. 12 months.

4. Which of the following presents the greatest risk to the child with hemophilia? *(619)*
   1. Hematuria
   2. Hemarthrosis
   3. Intracranial bleeding
   4. Anemia

5. Signs and symptoms that might indicate that a child has idiopathic thrombocytopenic purpura include: *(620)*
   1. headaches and hematuria.
   2. anemia and purpura.
   3. petechiae and purpura.
   4. hematuria and petechiae.

6. The diagnostic test that confirms a diagnosis of leukemia is a(n): *(621)*
   1. lumbar puncture.
   2. bone marrow aspiration.
   3. complete blood count.
   4. x-ray of the bones.

7. When caring for a child on steroid therapy, it is important to seek immediate medical attention if the child: *(622)*
   1. vomits.
   2. develops a fever.
   3. skips a meal.
   4. gains weight.

8. Children with Hodgkin's disease usually present with a(n): *(619)*
   1. rapid weight loss.
   2. painless cervical neck lump.
   3. enlarged abdomen.
   4. high fever.

9. Children with hemophilia should avoid: *(614)*
   1. swimming.
   2. salicylates.
   3. citrus fruits.
   4. analgesics.

10. Children with sickle cell trait: *(614)*
    1. have a 10% chance of developing the disease.
    2. have a 25% chance of developing the disease.
    3. have a 50% chance of developing the disease.
    4. will not develop the disease.

11. An appropriate nursing intervention for the child admitted to the hospital in sickle cell crisis would be to: *(616)*
    1. apply ice to painful areas.
    2. encourage the child to ambulate.
    3. provide foods high in iron at meals.
    4. monitor the child's response to analgesics.

12. Immediate nursing care of a child with hemophilia who has hemarthrosis includes: *(618)*
    1. application of heat.
    2. active and passive range-of-motion exercises.
    3. immobilization of the area.
    4. withholding factor VIII.

13. The greatest concern of a nurse caring for a child with ITP is: *(619)*
    1. noncompliance with aspirin therapy.
    2. a reaction to platelets.
    3. injuries that might initiate bleeding.
    4. development of a secondary bacterial infection.

14. Anxiety can be decreased in both the family and the child who has cancer by: *(630)*
    1. not telling the child that he or she has cancer.
    2. explaining all procedures before they are done.
    3. placing the child with an older child who has the same diagnosis.
    4. discouraging the child and parents from discussing the issue of death.

15. A common childhood disease that can have devastating effects on an immunosuppressed child is: *(621)*
    1. measles.
    2. chickenpox.
    3. rubella.
    4. nasopharyngitis.

16. Nursing care of an adolescent with cancer who is refusing to cooperate with treatment should include: *(626)*
    1. asking the parents to make the adolescent cooperate.
    2. allowing the adolescent to make some choices.
    3. withholding favorite foods until the behavior changes.
    4. restricting visitors until the behavior is modified.

17. What would be the initial nursing action when a child receiving a transfusion of packed red blood cells complains of chills and back pain? *(622)*
    1. Reduce the infusion rate.
    2. Take the child's blood pressure.
    3. Administer Benadryl as ordered.
    4. Discontinue the transfusion.

Student Name _____

CROSSWORD PUZZLE

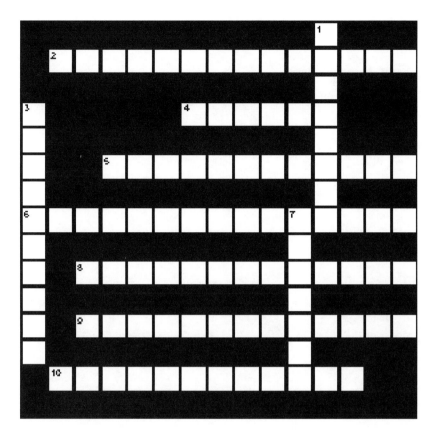

Across

2. Regulates the rate of RBC production *(610)*
4. A reduction in the size of RBCs or in amount of circulating hemoglobin *(612)*
5. Bleeding into a joint cavity *(618)*
6. Enlargement of lymph nodes *(610)*
8. Deposit of iron into organs and tissues of the body *(616)*
9. Type of sickle cell crisis caused by obstruction to blood flow by abnormally shaped cells *(615)*
10. Enlargement of the spleen *(611)*

Down

1. Raised ecchymosis *(619)*
3. A physician who specializes in treating cancer *(619)*
7. Large petechiae *(611)*

CHAPTER 27

The Child with a Gastrointestinal Condition

LEARNING ACTIVITIES

1. Match the terms in the left column with their definitions on the right (a–g).

   _____ Homeostasis *(647)*
   _____ Incarcerated *(640)*
   _____ Inguinal hernia *(640)*
   _____ Pica *(656)*
   _____ Projectile vomiting *(636)*
   _____ Pyloromyotomy *(636)*
   _____ Plumbism *(656)*

   a. Protrusion of part of the intestine through the umbilical ring
   b. Constricted hernia
   c. Eating nonfood items
   d. Operation to correct pyloric stenosis
   e. State of equilibrium of the body
   f. Vomiting in which the stomach contents are forcibly ejected
   g. Lead poisoning

2. List four of the possible common tests used to diagnose gastrointestinal disorders. *(633)*

   a. _____

   b. _____

   c. _____

   d. _____

3. The infant with tracheoesophageal fistula will _____ and _____ when the first feeding is given. *(635)*

4. Define *pyloric stenosis*. *(636)*

   _____

   _____

5. A complication of the vomiting associated with pyloric stenosis is _____ _____. *(636)*

6. Describe the progression of feeding after postoperative correction of pyloric stenosis. *(636)*

_____

_____

_____

_____

_____

7. Celiac disease is the leading _____ problem in children. *(638)*

8. Gluten is found in _____, _____, _____, and _____
_____. *(638)*

9. Stools in the child with celiac disease are _____, _____, and
_____. *(638)*

10. The earliest sign of Hirschsprung's disease is failure to pass meconium stools within _____ to
_____ hours after birth. *(639)*

11. Hirschsprung's disease is treated _____. It may be necessary for the infant to
have a _____ temporarily. *(639)*

12. Tap water enemas are never given to children because they can lead to _____
and _____. *(639)*

13. Describe the initial onset of intussusception. *(640)*

_____

_____

_____

14. Treatment of choice for intussusception is reduction through the use of a _____
_____. *(640)*

15. The most common congenital malformation of the gastrointestinal tract is _____
_____. *(640)*

16. Surgical repair of a hernia is called a _____. *(641)*

17. The priority concern for the infant with gastroenteritis is preventing _____
_____. *(663)*

18. Identify three nursing interventions for an infant hospitalized for gastroenteritis. *(663)*

a. _____

b. _____

c. _____

Student Name_____

19. Persistent vomiting can result in _____ and
_____. *(641)*

20. To prevent aspiration of vomitus after feeding, an infant should be placed in what position? *(641)*

_____

21. What would be included in the nurse's documentation for a child who is vomiting? *(641)*

a. _____

b. _____

c. _____

d. _____

e. _____

f. _____

g. _____

22. Define *gastroesophageal reflux. (642)* _____
_____

23. After a feeding, an infant with gastroesophageal reflux disease should be placed in which position? *(642)*

_____

24. Signs and symptoms of dehydration in the infant with diarrhea include: *(643)*

a. _____

b. _____

c. _____

d. _____

25. A 6-year-old child has mild diarrhea. How would the nurse advise the child's parents about fluid and food intake? *(643)*

_____

26. Name three high-fiber foods to recommend to an older child who is experiencing constipation. *(643)*

a. _____

b. _____

c. _____

27. In children under age 2, a greater percentage of body water is contained in the
_____ compartment. *(643)*

28. _____ is the greatest threat to life in isotonic dehydration. *(648)*

29. Failure to thrive (FTT) describes infants and children who _____
_____. *(649)*

30. Kwashiorkor results from a severe deficiency of _____ in the child's diet. *(650)*

31. List three signs and symptoms of rickets. *(651)*

    a. _____

    b. _____

    c. _____

32. The decrease of incidence of rickets in the world is attributed to _____
_____. *(651)*

33. Scurvy results from a deficiency of foods containing _____ in the diet. To
prevent scurvy, the nurse would encourage parents to include _____
and _____ in the child's diet. *(651)*

Answer as either true (T) or false (F).

34. Vomiting begins before abdominal pain with appendicitis. *(651)* _____

35. Fever is a reliable sign of appendicitis in children. *(651)* _____

36. Abdominal pain associated with appendicitis is localized in the right lower quadrant. *(651)* _____

37. The child with appendicitis may exhibit guarding and rebound tenderness when the nurse performs an
abdominal assessment. *(651)* _____

38. How is Nystatin applied to the mouth of a child with thrush? *(652)*

_____

39. What is the most common sign of pinworms? *(652)*

_____

40. Describe the treatment of pinworms. *(652-653)*

_____

_____

_____

_____

41. The goals in the treatment of poisoning are: *(653)*

    a. _____

    b. _____

    c. _____

    d. _____

Student Name _____

42. Activated charcoal should not be given with _____ because it will neutralize both, rendering both ineffective in the treatment of poisoning. *(653)*

43. An overdose of acetaminophen can result in _____ damage. *(654)*

44. The primary source of lead poisoning is _____. *(656)*

45. Lead poisoning can have a lasting effect on the _____ system. *(656)*

46. Match each type of dehydration with its definition (a–c).

    _____   Hypotonic *(648)*
    _____   Hypertonic *(648)*
    _____   Isotonic *(648)*

    a.   Loss of more electrolytes than water
    b.   Loss of equal amounts of water and electrolytes
    c.   Loss of more water than electrolytes

47. Interpret the following arterial blood gas values to determine the acid-base imbalance. *(649)*

    Acid-Base Imbalance

    a.   _____   pH 7.32 $PaCO_2$ 37 HCO_3 20

    b.   _____   pH 7.48 $PaCO_2$ 49 HCO_3 24

THINKING CRITICALLY

1. You are speaking to a parent whose child has mild diarrhea. The parent explains that she has been giving the child a BRAT diet. Is this an appropriate intervention? If not, what will you recommend for this child?

2. You are caring for a child who drank a poisonous substance. What feelings might the child's parents be having? How can you assist the parents?

CASE STUDY

1. Six-month-old Amber is diagnosed as failing to thrive. Amber's mother is a single parent who does not work outside the home. Neighbors report that they often hear Amber crying and that her mother seldom holds her. They also report that Amber's mother has related to them that being a mother is not what she thought it would be.
    a.   List some of the signs of failure to thrive.
    b.   What treatment might be implemented?
    c.   How would you involve Amber's mother in her care?
    d.   Discuss your feelings toward parents who neglect their children.

APPLYING KNOWLEDGE

1. Observe an endoscopy.

2. Use Figure 27-1 in the textbook to label the following.
   a. esophagus
   b. stomach
   c. pancreas
   d. liver
   e. gallbladder
   f. small intestine
   g. large intestine
   h. rectum

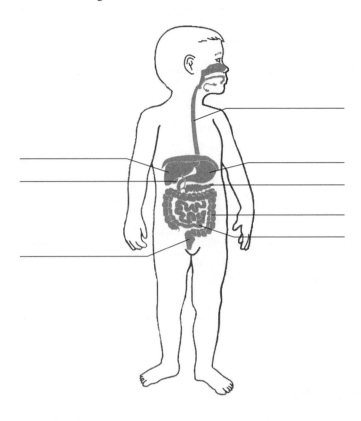

3. Develop a teaching plan related to poison prevention.

4. Develop a teaching plan related to caring for a child with diarrhea.

REVIEW QUESTIONS

1. Which diagnostic test permits visualization of the upper GI tract? *(633)*
   1. Colonoscopy
   2. Sigmoidoscopy
   3. Endoscopy
   4. Proctoscopy

2. Children with failure to thrive fall below the _____ percentile in weight and height on growth charts. *(650)*
   1. 3rd
   2. 6th
   3. 10th
   4. 15th

3. Which approach might best support maternal attachment when caring for a child with failure to thrive? *(650)*
   1. Point out areas where the mother needs improvement.
   2. Send the mother to a parenting class.
   3. Encourage the mother to participate in the child's care.
   4. Leave the room when the mother visits.

Student Name_____

4. Which signs and symptoms are characteristic of pinworms? *(652)*
   1. Diarrhea, itching, and fever
   2. Nausea, vomiting, and itching
   3. Nausea, vomiting, and weight loss
   4. Itching, irritability, and restlessness

5. Children with intussusception may have bowel movements containing blood and mucus and no feces. These are called: *(640)*
   1. currant jelly stools.
   2. mucoid stools.
   3. steatorrhea.
   4. occult blood stools.

6. A newborn's total body weight is about _____ water. *(646)*
   1. 77%
   2. 65%
   3. 55%
   4. 45%

7. Which action should the nurse take before adding potassium to a child's IV? *(648)*
   1. Take a baseline blood pressure.
   2. Determine if the child can tolerate oral fluids.
   3. Establish that the child is voiding.
   4. Place the child on a cardiac monitor.

8. The greatest threat to life in isotonic dehydration is: *(648)*
   1. hypervolemic shock.
   2. hypovolemic shock.
   3. respiratory acidosis.
   4. respiratory alkalosis.

9. The nurse taking a history from parents of an infant with pyloric stenosis would expect them to report the infant experienced which sign? *(636)*
   1. Constipation
   2. Projectile vomiting
   3. Diarrhea
   4. Anorexia

10. When a child has pinworms, the nurse knows that: *(653)*
    1. it is a sign of poor hygiene.
    2. the child will be hospitalized.
    3. any family member with symptoms should be treated.
    4. a warm stool specimen is sent to the lab.

11. Which information would the nurse give to parents of an infant with gastroesophageal reflux disease? *(642)*
    1. Feed the infant half-strength formula.
    2. Position in an infant seat after feeding.
    3. Increase the time between feedings.
    4. Place prone with the head elevated after feeding.

12. The nurse doing a newborn assessment knows the earliest sign of Hirschsprung's disease is: *(639)*
    1. failure to pass meconium.
    2. large, bulky, and frothy stools.
    3. acute, sudden diarrhea.
    4. ribbon-like stools.

13. The organ damaged by acetaminophen poisoning is the: *(654)*
    1. gallbladder.
    2. pancreas.
    3. liver.
    4. stomach.

14. The nurse would explain to parents that infants are more susceptible to accidental ingestion of foreign bodies because they are: *(657)*
    1. often left unattended.
    2. curious.
    3. constantly hungry.
    4. seeking parental attention.

15. The nurse was giving a newborn her first feeding when the baby started coughing and choking. This is indicative of which condition? *(634-635)*
    1. Celiac disease
    2. Enterocolitis
    3. Tracheoesophageal atresia
    4. Pyloric stenosis

16. A child appears apathetic and weak. His growth is below normal for his age. There is a white streak in the child's hair. The nurse recognizes these signs as characteristic of: *(651)*
    1. rickets.
    2. scurvy.
    3. gastroesophageal reflux.
    4. kwashiorkor.

17. Which statement indicates to the nurse that a parent understands information about prevention of lead poisoning? *(656)*
    1. "I give my child juice in an earthenware cup."
    2. "I use azarcon when my child has empacho."
    3. "My son would rather eat paint chips than cookies."
    4. "I wash any fresh fruit before giving it to my children."

18. A child's arterial blood gas results are: pH 7.30, $PaCO_2$ 31, HCO_3 25. The nurse determines the child is experiencing which acid-base imbalance? *(649)*
    1. Respiratory acidosis
    2. Respiratory alkalosis
    3. Metabolic acidosis
    4. Respiratory acidosis

28 The Child with a Genitourinary Condition

Student Name _____

Answer Key: Textbook page references are provided as a guide for answering these questions. A complete answer key was provided for your instructor.

LEARNING ACTIVITIES

1. Match the terms in the left column with their definitions on the right (a–j).

   _____ Cystitis *(664)*

   _____ Frequency *(662)*

   _____ Hydrocele *(669)*

   _____ Hypospadias *(662)*

   _____ Oliguria *(662)*

   _____ Phimosis *(662)*

   _____ Polyuria *(662)*

   _____ Pyelonephritis *(664)*

   _____ Urgency *(662)*

   _____ Vesicoureteral reflux *(664)*

   a. Backward flow of urine into the ureters
   b. Abnormal number of voidings in a short period of time
   c. Inflammation of the bladder
   d. Infection of the kidney substance and pelvis
   e. Excessive amount of fluid in the scrotal sac
   f. Decreased urinary output
   g. Narrowing of the preputial opening of the foreskin
   h. Urge to void but unable to do so
   i. Congenital defect in which the urinary meatus is not at the end of the penis but on the lower shaft
   j. Increased urinary output

2. List five tests used to determine the cause of urinary dysfunction. *(661)*

   a. _____

   b. _____

   c. _____

   d. _____

   e. _____

Answer as either true (T) or false (F).

3. The newborn's kidneys function immaturely. *(659, 660)* _____

4. There is an unexplained relationship between low-set ears and anomalies of the urinary tract. *(659)*

   _____

5. Phimosis is normal in newborn males and usually disappears by the time a boy is 3 years old. *(662)*
    _____

6. The optimal time for surgical repair of hypospadias and epispadias is in the late preschool period. *(662)*
    _____

7. Surgical repair of exstrophy of the bladder is done in the first 2 days of life. *(663)* _____

8. Distention of the renal pelvis due to an obstruction is referred to as _____
    _____. *(664)*

9. How would the nurse assess a child for bladder distention? *(664)*

    _____

    _____

10. List four of the possible reasons why urinary tract infections are more common in girls than in boys.
    (664)

    a. _____

    b. _____

    c. _____

    d. _____

11. Compare the signs and symptoms of a urinary tract infection in infants with those in older children.
    (665)

    Infant   *Older Child*

    a. _____   _____

    b. _____   _____

    c. _____   _____

    d. _____   _____

12. What laboratory test is done to confirm a diagnosis of urinary tract infection? *(665)*

    _____

13. What classification of medication is used to treat a urinary tract infection in a 4-year-old child? *(665)*

    _____

14. The characteristic sign of nephrotic syndrome is _____. *(665)*

15. Edema associated with nephrotic syndrome usually occurs first around the _____
    and _____. *(665)*

16. The nurse would expect a urinalysis of a child with nephrotic syndrome to reveal massive _____
    _____. *(665)*

17. What is the treatment of choice for nephrotic syndrome? *(665)*

_____

18. List three types of skin care that might be given to a child with nephrotic syndrome. *(667)*

a. _____

b. _____

c. _____

19. When observing the urine of a child with nephrotic syndrome, the nurse should note: *(667)*

a. _____

b. _____

c. _____

d. _____

20. The child receiving treatment for nephrotic syndrome is at risk for _____.
    (665, 668)

21. Acute glomerulonephritis is thought to be a(n) _____
    reaction caused by _____. *(668)*

22. List four nursing interventions that would be appropriate for the child who has acute glomerulonephri-
    tis. *(668-669)*

a. _____

b. _____

c. _____

d. _____

23. Foods high in _____ are restricted when a child with acute glomerulonephritis is oligu-
    ric. *(669)*

24. What organ is affected by Wilms' tumor? *(669)* _____

25. What is involved in the treatment of Wilms' tumor? *(669)*

a. _____

b. _____

c. _____

26. What precaution is taken in a child with a Wilms' tumor to prevent spread of the disease? *(669)*

_____

_____

Answer as either true (T) or false (F).

27. Cryptorchidism can affect the development of secondary sex characteristics. *(671)* _____

28. Cryptorchidism increases the risk of testicular cancer in adulthood. *(672)* _____

THINKING CRITICALLY

1. A child you are caring for is in renal failure as a result of chronic glomerulonephritis. She is being evaluated for a kidney transplant. Use the library to research this topic. Include in your information the selection process, procedure, risks, expense, recovery, and maintenance.

CASE STUDY

1. Three-year-old Tucker is hospitalized with nephrotic syndrome. Tucker is pale, lethargic, anorexic, and has generalized edema.
   a. Tucker is put on steroid therapy. What are three nursing interventions associated with his treatment?
   b. Plan a menu for Tucker for one day using the nutritional requirements necessary for his recovery.
   c. Tucker likes to lie on his stomach. When you change his position, he is irritable and his mother objects. What would you tell his mother?

APPLYING KNOWLEDGE

1. Use Figure 28-1 in the textbook to label the following.
   a. kidney
   b. ureter
   c. urinary bladder
   d. urethra

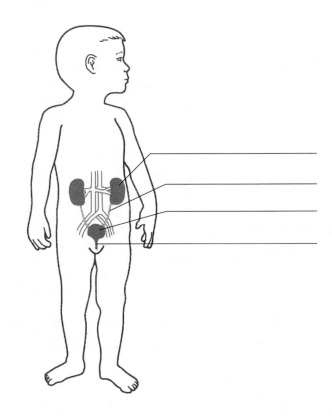

Student Name_____

2. While in the clinical area, collect a urine specimen from an infant and a toddler.

3. Measure abdominal girth on a child with ascites.

4. Keep an intake and output record on a child with a genitourinary condition.

REVIEW QUESTIONS

1. The nurse planning care for a child with nephrotic syndrome knows the classification of medication used to reduce edema in nephrotic syndrome is: *(665)*
   1. diuretics.
   2. antibiotics.
   3. analgesics.
   4. steroids.

2. An expected outcome for a child with nephrotic syndrome is the prevention of: *(667)*
   1. skin breakdown.
   2. an antigen–antibody reaction.
   3. pathologic fractures.
   4. urinary stasis.

3. Which statement indicates to the nurse that a parent understands information about hypospadias? *(662)*
   1. "This defect must be corrected in the first few days of life."
   2. "Fertility will most likely be reduced."
   3. "The condition may resolve by the first birthday."
   4. "Surgical repair is usually performed by age 18 months."

4. Which instructions would the nurse give parents about activity restrictions for a child with acute glomerulonephritis? *(668)*
   1. No restrictions on activity
   2. Remain on bed rest for 2 weeks
   3. Limited activity until gross hematuria subsides
   4. Avoid team sports if neutropenic

5. The nurse would assess a child with acute glomerulonephritis for which the presence of: *(668)*
   1. urinary frequency.
   2. petechiae.
   3. hypotension.
   4. hypertension.

6. Wilms' tumors are often discovered when: *(669)*
   1. children enter school.
   2. the child has flank pain.
   3. blood is noted in the urine.
   4. a routine physical is given.

7. A parent reports her son's urethral opening is located on the undersurface of the penis. The nurse recognizes the child has which genitourinary condition? *(662)*
   1. Hydrocele
   2. Phimosis
   3. Hypospadias
   4. Cryptorchidism

8. What information would the nurse include when teaching young girls about preventing urinary tract infections? *(665)*
   1. Wear nylon underwear.
   2. Void only when their bladder is full.
   3. Limit fluids after 8:00 PM.
   4. Wipe themselves from the front to the back.

9. The etiology of acute glomerulonephritis is thought to be a(n): *(668)*
   1. antigen–antibody reaction.
   2. autoimmune disease.
   3. primary disease.
   4. infectious disease.

10. The nurse assessing urinary output for a child with acute glomerulonephritis would expect urine to be: *(668)*
    1. straw-colored.
    2. smoky brown.
    3. cloudy and concentrated.
    4. yellow with many mucous shreds.

11. Which is a sign of a urinary tract infection in a 6-year-old child? *(665)*
    1. Proteinuria
    2. Perineal rash
    3. Hematuria
    4. Pain during micturition

12. The nurse is caring for a child who has a ureterostomy. With this urinary diversion the nurse is aware: *(664)*
    1. urine drains from the pelvis of the kidney through a tube.
    2. an opening was created into the bladder between the umbilicus and pubis.
    3. ureters are surgically implanted to outside the abdominal wall.
    4. a tube into the bladder above the pubis provides urinary drainage.

13. Children receiving steroids should be: *(665)*
    1. placed on antibiotics before there are signs of an infection.
    2. isolated from other children receiving steroids.
    3. monitored closely for signs of infection.
    4. taken off the medication after 1 week.

14. When weighing diapers on a gram scale, the conversion from grams to milliliters is: *(667)*
    1. 1 g = 2.5 ml.
    2. 1 g = 1 ml.
    3. 1 g = 0.5 ml.
    4. 1 g = 0.25 ml.

15. While the child with nephrotic syndrome is being treated, he or she should not receive: *(668)*
    1. antihistamines.
    2. immunizations.
    3. diuretics.
    4. analgesics.

Student Name _____

16. While caring for a child with glomerulonephritis, the nurse observes a rise in the child's blood pressure. What is the most appropriate nursing action? *(668)*
    1. Document the change.
    2. Recheck the blood pressure in 2 hours.
    3. Notify the physician.
    4. Restrict sodium and fluid intake.

17. What is an acceptable urine output for a 2-year-old child weighing 27 pounds? *(662)*
    1. 10 ml/hour
    2. 30 ml/hour
    3. 50 ml/hour
    4. 70 ml/hour

18. What nursing action would be avoided when caring for a child diagnosed with Wilms' tumor? *(669)*
    1. Measuring urinary output
    2. Monitoring blood pressure
    3. Abdominal palpation
    4. Auscultation of lungs sounds

19. A parent tells the nurse, "My child is going to have a test that takes an x-ray before and while he is urinating." The child is scheduled for which diagnostic study? *(661)*
    1. Voiding cystourethrography
    2. Cystoscopy
    3. Cystometrogram
    4. Uroflow study

CROSSWORD PUZZLE

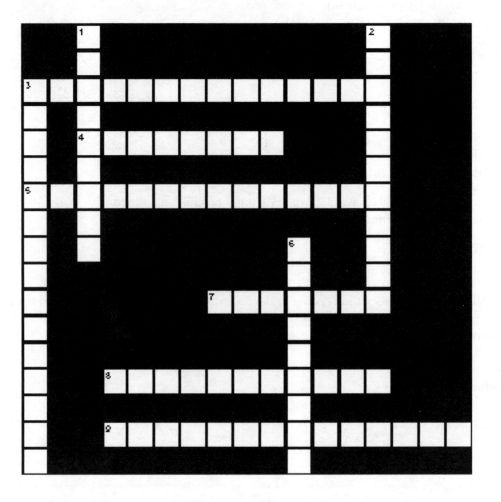

Across

3. Distention of the renal pelvis caused by obstruction *(664)*
4. Decreased urinary output *(662)*
5. Infection of the kidney and renal pelvis *(664)*
7. Urge to void but inability to do so *(662)*
8. Absolute neutrophil count below 1000/mm³ *(665)*
9. Undescended testicle *(671)*

Down

1. Excessive amount of fluid in the sac that surrounds the testicle *(669)*
2. Surgical opening into the bladder between the umbilicus and pubis *(664)*
3. Decreased level of protein in the blood *(665)*
6. Abnormal number of voidings in a short period *(662)*

CHAPTER 29

The Child with a Skin Condition

Answer Key: Textbook page references are provided as a guide for answering these questions. A complete answer key was provided for your instructor.

LEARNING ACTIVITIES

1. Match the terms in the left column with their definitions on the right (a–j).

   _____ Comedo *(679)*
   _____ Debridement *(690)*
   _____ Exanthem *(675)*
   _____ Heterograft *(690)*
   _____ Homograft *(690)*
   _____ Isograft *(690)*
   _____ Miliaria *(677)*
   _____ Pruritus *(677)*
   _____ Strawberry nevus *(676)*
   _____ Wheal *(676)*

   a. Benign hemangioma that disappears without treatment
   b. Graft tissue from a source other than human
   c. Removal of dried crusts
   d. Graft tissue from cadavers
   e. Irregular red, raised area associated with allergic reactions
   f. Plug of keratin, sebum, and bacteria
   g. Skin rash
   h. Graft from the patient's identical twin
   i. Itching
   j. Rash caused by excess body heat and moisture

2. Name three tests used in diagnosing skin conditions. *(675)*

   a. _____

   b. _____

   c. _____

3. Name three of the possible characteristics of skin lesions. *(675)*

   a. _____

   b. _____

   c. _____

4. What is miliaria? *(677)*

   _____

5. How can intertrigo be prevented? *(678)* _____

    _____

6. How would the nurse advise parents about the treatment for an infant who has seborrheic dermatitis? *(678)*

    _____

    _____

    _____

7. How can diaper dermatitis be prevented? *(678)*

    _____

    _____

8. Briefly describe the pathology of acne. *(678-679)*

    _____

    _____

9. Patients taking vitamin A should avoid _____. *(679)*

10. The main concern of anyone taking Accutane is to _____

    _____. *(679)*

11. A medication that may reduce viral shedding and hasten healing of herpes simplex type 1 infection is

    _____. *(680)*

12. Eczema is indicative of _____. *(680)*

13. Allergens enter the body of the child with eczema through: *(680)*

    a. _____

    b. _____

    c. _____

    d. _____

14. Describe the application of ointment to the skin of a child with eczema. *(679, 680)*

    _____

    _____

    _____

15. The organism responsible for causing scalded skin syndrome is _____. *(681)*

16. What is impetigo? *(684)* _____

    _____

Student Name_____

17. How can impetigo be prevented? *(684)*

_____

_____

18. Describe the treatment of impetigo. *(684)*

_____

_____

_____

19. Identify the body parts affected in the following tinea infections. *(684-685)*

    a.   Tinea capitis: _____

    b.   Tinea corporis: _____

    c.   Tinea pedis: _____

    d.   Tinea cruris: _____

20. Describe the treatment of tinea capitis. *(684)*

_____

_____

_____

Answer as either true (T) or false (F).

21. Tinea occurs when fungus invades the hair, the stratum corneum layer of the skin, or the nails. *(684)*
_____

22. Tinea infections are not contagious to others. *(684)* _____

23. Tinea pedis heals more quickly if the affected area is kept warm and moist. *(685)* _____

24. The main symptom of pediculosis is _____. *(685)*

25. The most common form of pediculosis infestation is _____. *(685)*

26. What are scabies? *(685)*

_____

_____

27. List the four types of burns. *(687)*

    a. _____

    b. _____

    c. _____

    d. _____

28. When a child is burned by fire near the face, assessing for _____ and _____ is a priority. *(687)*

29. The severity of a burn depends on the _____, _____, and _____ of involvement. *(687)*

30. Match the burn classification with the correct description (a–c).

    _____ First degree *(688)*   a. Blistered, moist, pink, or red; painful
    _____ Second degree *(688)*   b. Tough, leathery, dry; painless to touch
    _____ Third degree *(688)*   c. Skin red but blanches easily and refills quickly; painful

31. Indications of an inhalation problem in a patient who has been burned include: *(689)*

    a. _____

    b. _____

    c. _____

    d. _____

32. If eschar from burns on the trunk inhibits respirations, an _____ is made in order to prevent restriction of chest movement. *(689)*

33. Urine output is observed _____ in a burn patient. *(689)*

34. What is the rationale for inserting a nasogastric tube into a burn patient? *(689)*

    _____

    _____

35. Describe how a burn wound is dressed. *(690)*

    _____

    _____

    _____

    _____

    _____

Student Name_____

36. Describe how protective isolation is instituted with a burn patient. *(691)*

_____

_____

_____

_____

_____

37. List the signs and symptoms of infection in a burn patient. *(692)*

   a. _____

   b. _____

   c. _____

   d. _____

   e. _____

38. What type of diet should a burn patient be given? *(692)*

_____

_____

_____

39. Analgesics are administered _____ painful procedures, such as dressing changes. *(692)*

40. The school nurse is talking with children about preventing frostbite. What should be included in the nurse's explanation about dressing for outdoor activities? *(693)*

_____

_____

THINKING CRITICALLY

1. Use the nursing process to prepare care for a 9-year-old child who was admitted to the hospital with full-thickness burns of the chest and arms 2 days ago. He is burned over 15% of his body. His treatment plan includes an IV, reverse isolation, occlusive dressings with Silvadene to the wound, regular diet with high-protein feedings between meals, and morphine for pain. What do you consider to be the four most important nursing diagnoses? State expected outcomes of care and nursing interventions for one nursing diagnosis. Compare your care plan with others.

CASE STUDIES

1. Stacey, a 17-year-old teenager diagnosed with acne vulgaris, is prescribed Accutane because other medications have not been effective.
   a. What can the nurse tell Stacey about the side effects of Accutane?
   b. Stacey asks if there is anything she can do with her diet to improve the acne. What should the nurse tell her?
   c. What are some topical preparations that could be recommended for Stacey's acne?

2. Ten-month-old Taylor is admitted to the hospital with a diagnosis of atopic dermatitis. His face, arms, and legs are erythematous and are covered with vesicles, some of which have crusted over. The physician's orders are Isomil formula, continuous wet compresses of Burow's solution to extremities, cut fingernails, and place in private room.
   a. What is infantile eczema (atopic dermatitis)?
   b. What does the order for Isomil have to do with Taylor's diagnosis?
   c. Describe how the nurse will prepare the wet compresses, their purpose, documentation, and any special care that will be taken while they are on Taylor.
   d. What are some of the psychologic needs of a child with eczema?
   e. Taylor is irritable and continually attempts to scratch his arms and legs. What can the nurse do to soothe him?

APPLYING KNOWLEDGE

1. When you are in the clinical setting, read the charts and find a description of skin on:
   a. an admission assessment.
   b. a child with a skin disorder.
   c. a child with a burn.

REVIEW QUESTIONS

1. Which of the following skin conditions is *not* contagious? *(680)*
   1. Impetigo
   2. *Staphylococcus aureus* infection
   3. Infantile eczema
   4. Pediculosis

2. What information would the nurse give to parents about the treatment of pediculosis capitis? *(685)*
   1. All family members must be treated.
   2. Wash the child's hair with hydrogen peroxide.
   3. Apply prescription lotion to the entire body.
   4. Use a fine-toothed comb to remove nits.

3. The nurse determines a parent understands instructions when she tells the nurse first-aid treatment of a partial-thickness burn should include: *(688)*
   1. application of butter.
   2. immersion in cold water.
   3. elevation of the involved area.
   4. breaking the blisters.

Student Name_____

4. A full-thickness burn can best be described as: *(688)*
   1. red with good refill, painful.
   2. mottled, red, dull white, painful.
   3. blistered, pink or red, painful.
   4. tough, leathery, painless to touch.

5. The nurse assessing a child with burns recognizes which finding as an early sign of sepsis? *(692)*
   1. Decreased pulse
   2. Erythema
   3. Elevated temperature
   4. Decreased blood pressure

6. A burn patient with cyanosis and charred lips may need a(n): *(689)*
   1. nasogastric tube.
   2. endotracheal tube.
   3. Foley catheter.
   4. throat culture.

7. The priority goal in the management of a severe burn is: *(689)*
   1. wound debridement.
   2. pain control.
   3. fluid replacement.
   4. airway maintenance.

8. The nurse would teach parents of a child with impetigo to be alert for signs of which complication? *(684)*
   1. Rheumatoid arthritis
   2. Nephritis
   3. Endocarditis
   4. Otitis media

9. The nurse would instruct an adolescent who is taking Accutane to avoid: *(679)*
   1. sun exposure.
   2. dairy products.
   3. pregnancy.
   4. strenuous exercise.

10. When inspecting children for pediculosis capitis, special attention should be paid to which area of the body? *(685)*
    1. Pubic area
    2. Hairline at the back of the neck
    3. Area around the forehead
    4. Underarms

11. A common manifestation of an allergy in a neonate is: *(680)*
    1. port wine stain.
    2. eczema.
    3. strawberry nevus.
    4. Mongolian spots.

12. What is the most appropriate nursing response to an adolescent who asks what she can do about her acne? *(679)*
    1. "Restrict the amount of chocolate and peanuts you eat."
    2. "Wash your face at least four times a day."
    3. "Get adequate rest and eat a well-balanced diet."
    4. "Stay out of the sun even if you are not on medication."

13. The nurse is caring for a child who received a skin graft from pigskin. This type of graft is called a(n): *(690)*
    1. homograft.
    2. heterograft.
    3. isograft.

14. A priority in changing the dressing of a burn patient is: *(692)*
    1. asking the parents to leave the room.
    2. medicating for pain prior to the procedure.
    3. limiting the number of dressing changes.
    4. doing the procedure in the child's room.

15. A child who has been burned eats only a small amount of the food on her tray. An appropriate nursing action would be to: *(692)*
    1. request an order to start an IV.
    2. insert a nasogastric tube for feeding.
    3. offer the child small, frequent feedings.
    4. leave the tray at the bedside longer.

16. Scabies are characterized by: *(685)*
    1. round, dry patches on the arms.
    2. intense itching.
    3. a purulent drainage.
    4. round lesions similar to chickenpox.

17. A topical ointment is prescribed for an infant with eczema. What instructions would the nurse provide to the parent about application of the medication? *(681)*
    1. Apply a generous amount of ointment to affected areas.
    2. Use a circular motion to massage the ointment into the skin.
    3. Keep the fingernails short to prevent scratching the infant.
    4. For best absorption, apply ointment after bathing the child.

30 The Child with a Metabolic Condition

LEARNING ACTIVITIES

1. Match the terms in the left column with their definitions on the right (a–g).

   _____ Glycosuria *(700)*
   _____ Hormones *(695)*
   _____ Hyperglycemia *(700)*
   _____ Hypoglycemia *(707)*
   _____ Kussmaul respirations *(701)*
   _____ Polydipsia *(700)*
   _____ Polyphagia *(700)*

   a. Excessive thirst
   b. Constant hunger
   c. Increased glucose in the blood
   d. Glucose in the urine
   e. Type of respirations seen in diabetic ketoacidosis
   f. Decreased glucose in the blood
   g. Chemical substances produced by glands

2. Identify five early signs of inborn errors of metabolism in a newborn. *(695)*

   a. _____

   b. _____

   c. _____

   d. _____

   e. _____

3. The pattern of inheritance for inborn errors of metabolism is generally _____
   _____. *(696)*

4. _____ testing and _____ counseling
   have markedly decreased the occurrence of Tay-Sachs disease. *(697)*

5. List five manifestations of hypothyroidism. *(697)*

   a. _____

   b. _____

   c. _____

   d. _____

   e. _____

6. What is essential to prevent sequelae associated with congenital hypothyroidism? *(697)*

   _____

7. What information would the nurse give to parents about medication for the treatment of hypothyroidism? *(697)*

   _____

   _____

8. Describe the pathophysiology of diabetes insipidus. *(697)*

   _____

9. The initial signs of diabetes insipidus are _____ and
   _____. *(697)*

10. What would the nurse teach parents about administering DDAVP nasal spray to a child with diabetes insipidus? *(698)*

    _____

11. Describe the pathophysiology of diabetes mellitus. *(698)*

    _____

    _____

    _____

    _____

12. Type 1 diabetes mellitus is considered to be a(n) _____ disease. *(699)*

13. Type 2 diabetes mellitus involves a _____ to insulin. *(699)*

14. The onset of type 1 diabetes mellitus is increased in pubescent children. Give two possible causes of this increase. *(699)*

    a. _____

    _____

    b. _____

    _____

Student Name_____

15. What are the three "Ps" of type 1 diabetes mellitus? *(700)*

    a. _____

    b. _____

    c. _____

16. What is the most reliable test to diagnose diabetes mellitus? *(728)*

    _____

17. What test measures glycemic levels over a period of months? *(700)*

    _____

18. List the three goals of treatment in type 1 diabetes mellitus. *(701)*

    a. _____

    b. _____

    c. _____

19. Children with diabetes mellitus have problems associated with their stage of growth and development. Give at least one example of a problem for each age group. *(701)*

    a. Infant _____

    _____

    b. Toddler _____

    _____

    c. Preschool child_____

    _____

    d. School-age child_____

    _____

    e. Adolescent _____

    _____

20. List three goals of nutritional management for the child with type 1 diabetes mellitus. *(704)*

    a. _____

    _____

    b. _____

    _____

    c. _____

    _____

21. The standard form of insulin is _____. *(705)*

22. Describe insulin injection site rotation. *(705-706)*

   _____

   _____

   _____

   _____

   _____

23. List three reasons why a child is more prone to insulin shock than an adult. *(707)*

   a. _____

   b. _____

   c. _____

24. What is the immediate treatment for a child suspected of having an insulin reaction? *(707)*

   _____

   _____

25. _____ may be given for the treatment of severe hypoglycemia. *(707)*

26. Explain the Somogyi phenomenon. *(707)*

   _____

   _____

   _____

27. List two precautions in the foot care of a child with diabetes. *(709)*

   a. _____

   b. _____

28. When a child with diabetes plans to travel, what should be done prior to and during the trip? *(710)*

   a. _____

   b. _____

   c. _____

   d. _____

Student Name _____

29. Match each sign or symptom with its cause. (Causes may be used more than once.)

_____ Fruity breath *(701)*
_____ Headache *(701)*
_____ Diaphoretic *(701)*
_____ Abdominal pain *(701)*
_____ Tremors *(701)*
_____ Deep, rapid respirations *(701)*

a. Hypoglycemia
b. Hyperglycemia

Answer as either true (T) or false (F).

30. The symptoms of diabetes mellitus appear more slowly in children. *(700)* _____

31. Exercise lowers blood glucose levels. *(708)* _____

32. Water intake should be limited for the child with diabetes insipidus. *(698)* _____

33. Children with type I diabetes mellitus require special foods. *(704)* _____

34. The child with type I diabetes mellitus is able to participate in almost all sports activities. *(708)* _____

35. If left untreated, congenital hypothyroidism can result in mental retardation. *(697)* _____

36. When mixing insulin, the nurse draws up the longer-acting insulin into the syringe first. *(706)* _____

37. Human insulin manufactured by biosynthesis is the treatment of choice for type 1 diabetes mellitus. *(706)* _____

THINKING CRITICALLY

1. Plot a curve showing the peaks and duration of action for a child who is receiving a combination of regular and NPH insulin at 7:30 AM and 5:30 PM.

CASE STUDY

1. Anne, a 16 years old, is newly diagnosed with type 1 diabetes mellitus. She is a cheerleader and plays basketball. Since her diagnosis, Anne's parents are constantly with Anne and are very protective of her.
   a. Anne asks if she has to eat special foods. What would the nurse Anne about nutritional management of diabetes mellitus?
   b. Anne asks if she can still play basketball and remain a cheerleader. What should the nurse tell her about these activities?
   c. Anne becomes very impatient with her mother and accuses her of hovering. How can emotional turmoil have an effect on an adolescent with diabetes mellitus?
   d. How would the nurse respond to Anne when she asks, "How did I get diabetes?"

APPLYING KNOWLEDGE

1. While in the clinical area, teach a child or a parent to give insulin.

2. While in the clinical area, teach a family home glucose monitoring.

3. Care for a child in diabetic ketoacidosis.

REVIEW QUESTIONS

1. A child receives Lispro insulin before breakfast. She should eat her meal: *(707)*
   1. immediately.
   2. within 15 minutes.
   3. within 40 minutes.
   4. within 60 minutes.

2. Children can usually give their own insulin injections after the age of: *(705)*
   1. 7 years.
   2. 9 years.
   3. 11 years.
   4. 13 years.

3. An initial sign of diabetes insipidus is: *(697)*
   1. polyphagia.
   2. polydipsia.
   3. excessive perspiration.
   4. hyperglycemia.

4. What is the best food choice for the nurse to give to a child having an insulin reaction? *(707)*
   1. Orange juice
   2. Unsalted crackers
   3. Diet soda
   4. Apple slices

5. The nurse recognizes a sign of diabetic ketoacidosis is: *(701)*
   1. cold perspiration.
   2. decreased heart rate.
   3. deep, rapid respirations.
   4. slurred speech.

6. The most common concentration of insulin is: *(705)*
   1. U35 insulin.
   2. U40 insulin.
   3. U80 insulin.
   4. U100 insulin.

7. Which type of insulin is an intermediate-acting insulin? *(735)*
   1. Regular
   2. Lente
   3. Lantus
   4. Ultralente

8. The nurse determines a parent understands teaching about hypoglycemia when he identified which as a cause of hypoglycemia in children? *(707)*
   1. Eating too much food
   2. Using insufficient insulin
   3. Gastrointestinal Illness
   4. Poorly planned exercise

Student Name_____

9. The nurse recognizes a child with type 1 diabetes mellitus is having an insulin reaction when which sign occurs? *(701, 707)*
    1. Dry skin
    2. Flushed face
    3. Cold perspiration
    4. Increased thirst

10. Regular insulin is considered to be a(n): *(707)*
    1. rapid-acting insulin.
    2. intermediate-acting insulin.
    3. long-acting insulin.

11. A characteristic common to type 1 diabetes mellitus is that it: *(733)*
    1. is more common in preschool-age children.
    2. is often seen in obese individuals.
    3. always requires insulin.
    4. has few blood sugar fluctuations.

12. What information would the nurse include when speaking to expectant parents about Tay-Sachs Disease? *(696-697)*
    1. One parent passes the disease to the child.
    2. There is no known cause for this disease.
    3. There is a positive outcome if diagnosed before age 6 months.
    4. Carriers can be identified by a screening test.

13. The nurse would teach a child with type I diabetes mellitus to check urine for acetone when he: *(709)*
    1. is exercising.
    2. is sick.
    3. eats meals.
    4. has a growth spurt.

14. The nurse would explain to parents that screening infants for hypothyroidism is: *(697)*
    1. ordered for children of high-risk families.
    2. done on all infants at 6 months of age.
    3. done on all infants at birth.
    4. ineffective.

15. What information would the nurse include in teaching about thyroid hormone replacement for children with hypothyroidism? *(697)*
    1. It may cause excessive hair growth on the body.
    2. Medication is continued for the duration of the child's life.
    3. The full effect may not be reached for 3 months.
    4. Signs of overdosage include lethargy and constipation.

16. The nurse determines a parent of a child with diabetes insipidus requires additional teaching when she says a sign of water intoxication is: *(698)*
    1. polyuria.
    2. edema.
    3. nausea.
    4. lethargy.

17. The nurse teaching parents about type 2 diabetes mellitus would explain that it is associated with insulin: *(699)*
    1. overproduction.
    2. sensitivity.
    3. deficiency.
    4. resistance.

Student Name _____

The Child with a Communicable Disease

Answer Key: Textbook page references are provided as a guide for answering these questions. A complete answer key was provided for your instructor.

LEARNING ACTIVITIES

1. Match the terms in the left column with their definitions on the right (a–h).

   _____ Epidemic *(716)*

   _____ Erythema *(718)*

   _____ Fomite *(712)*

   _____ Incubation period *(712)*

   _____ Pandemic *(716)*

   _____ Prodromal period *(712)*

   _____ Vector *(716)*

   _____ Vesicle *(718)*

   a. Interval between the earliest symptoms and the appearance of the rash or fever
   b. Inanimate material that absorbs and transmits infection
   c. Insect or animal that carries and spreads a disease
   d. Sudden increase of a communicable disease in a localized area
   e. Diffused, reddened area on the skin
   f. Circular, reddened area on the skin that is elevated and contains fluid
   g. Worldwide high incidence of a communicable disease
   h. Time between invasion by a pathogen and the onset of symptoms

2. Define *communicable disease.* *(712)* _____

   _____

3. The incubation period for varicella is _____. *(713)*

4. How long is the child with varicella contagious? *(713)* _____

5. Describe the appearance of the child with fifth disease. *(713)*

   _____

6. List the manifestations of infectious mononucleosis. *(714)*

   a. _____

   b. _____

   c. _____

   d. _____

7. Identify three actions that can be taken to prevent Lyme disease. *(715)*

   a. _____

   b. _____

   c. _____

8. Careful _____ is basic and essential to contain infection. *(716)*

9. What is an opportunistic infection? *(717)*

   _____

   _____

10. A child developed a wound infection while he was hospitalized postoperatively. This is called a _____ infection. *(717)*

11. List three factors related to host resistance to disease. *(717)*

    a. _____

    b. _____

    c. _____

12. Vaccines provide _____ immunity to disease. *(717)*

13. A child received tetanus serum to prevent lockjaw. This is an example of _____ immunity. *(717)*

14. The Centers for Disease Control recommends _____ precautions for all patients. This involves _____ and _____ _____. *(718)*

15. When would the nurse use contact precautions? *(718)*

    _____

16. When would a child need expanded precautions? *(718)* _____

    _____

Student Name_____

17. Match the following terms with the correct description (a–e).

_____   Macule *(718)*

_____   Papule *(718)*

_____   Vesicle *(718)*

_____   Pustule *(718)*

_____   Scab *(718)*

   a.   Dried pustule covered with a crust

   b.   Circular, reddened area on the skin that is elevated and contains fluid

   c.   Circular, reddened area on the skin

   d.   Circular, reddened area on the skin that is elevated and contains pus

   e.   Circular, reddened area on the skin that is elevated

18. Why are immunizations not administered to infants under 2 months of age? *(719)* _____
_____

19. The _____ of vaccine administration influences the infant's response. *(720)*

20. _____ should be available on units where immunizations are given. *(720)*

21. List six contraindications to administration of a live virus vaccine. *(721)*

   a.   _____

   b.   _____

   c.   _____

   d.   _____

   e.   _____

   f.   _____

22. The occurrence of a sexually transmitted infection in a 9-year-old child suggests the possibility of
_____. *(724)*

23. List the three ways in which children can acquire the human immunodeficiency virus (HIV). *(725)*

   a.   _____

   b.   _____

   c.   _____

24. Identify three nursing diagnoses for a toddler with AIDS. *(726-728)*

   a.   _____

   b.   _____

   c.   _____

THINKING CRITICALLY

1. Four-month-old Orlando has come to the pediatrician's office for his well-child checkup. His mother tells you that Orlando's immunizations are up to date. Refer to the immunization schedule (Figure 31-6 in the textbook) to determine which immunizations he should receive at this visit.

2. You are asked to care for an adolescent with pelvic inflammatory disease. You know that she has been sexually active and has a history of STDs. Think about this situation and then write down your thoughts about this patient.

APPLYING KNOWLEDGE

1. Contact your local health department for information about educating the public about STDs. Request pamphlets and other written materials.

2. Assist nurses in a public health clinic to administer immunizations.

REVIEW QUESTIONS

1. Which disease does not require a routine immunization? *(722)*
    1. Chickenpox
    2. Smallpox
    3. Measles
    4. German measles

2. The period that refers to the initial stage of a disease between the earliest symptoms and the appearance of the rash or fever is the: *(712)*
    1. incubation period.
    2. infectious period.
    3. prodromal period.
    4. stage one period.

3. A child manifested signs and symptoms of RSV infection during a hospitalization for sickle cell crisis. This is referred to as a(n): *(717)*
    1. opportunistic infection.
    2. health-care associated infection.
    3. directly transmitted infection.
    4. pathognomonic infection.

4. A hospitalized child has varicella. The nurse would arrange for which type of infection precautions? *(718)*
    1. Large droplet infection precautions
    2. Airborne infection precautions
    3. Communicable disease precautions
    4. Indirect transmission precautions

Student Name _____

5. While inspecting a child's skin, the nurse observes a circular, reddened area that is elevated and contains fluid. The nurse would document this finding as a: *(718)*
   1. vesicle.
   2. pustule.
   3. macule.
   4. papule.

6. A parent asks the nurse she when her younger child will get chickenpox now that her oldest child contracted the illness. The nurse would explain the incubation period for chickenpox is: *(713)*
   1. 1–2 weeks.
   2. 2–3 weeks.
   3. 3–4 weeks.
   4. 4–5 weeks.

7. A child with pertussis would be placed in which type of isolation? *(718)*
   1. Droplet precautions
   2. Airborne precautions
   3. Contact precautions
   4. Expanded precautions

8. The most important nursing action in preventing the spread of infection is: *(716)*
   1. the administration of antibiotics.
   2. placing all children in private rooms.
   3. good handwashing.
   4. good nutrition.

9. The nurse observes Koplik's spots in the mouth of a child. This finding is associated with which communicable disease? *(713)*
   1. Chickenpox
   2. Rubella
   3. Rubeola
   4. Mumps

10. The risk of secondary infection in communicable diseases is reduced by: *(713)*
    1. giving all children antibiotics.
    2. keeping fingernails short.
    3. forcing fluids.
    4. isolating the child.

11. The disease that causes a "slapped cheek" appearance is: *(715)*
    1. Lyme disease.
    2. roseola.
    3. strep throat.
    4. fifth disease.

12. A child should receive the measles, mumps, rubella (MMR) vaccine at: *(722)*
    1. 4 months.
    2. 6 months.
    3. 15 months.
    4. 24 months.

13. If a vaccination series is interrupted: *(721)*
    1. the series must start over.
    2. it continues without restarting the entire series.
    3. the age of the child determines if the series must be restarted.
    4. the child must wait 6 months before restarting the series.

14. Which child should not receive a live virus vaccine? *(721)*
    1. Taking prednisone
    2. Has a sexually transmitted infection
    3. Was born prematurely
    4. Has a seizure disorder

CHAPTER 32

The Child with an Emotional or Behavioral Condition

Answer Key: Textbook page references are provided as a guide for answering these questions. A complete answer key was provided for your instructor.

LEARNING ACTIVITIES

1. Match the terms in the left column with their definitions on the right (a–f).

   _____ Gateway substances *(735)*
   _____ Milieu therapy *(731)*
   _____ Psychosomatic *(731)*
   _____ Suicidal attempt *(733)*
   _____ Suicidal gestures *(733)*
   _____ Suicidal ideation *(733)*

   a. Thoughts about suicide
   b. Attempt at a suicidal-type action that does not result in injury
   c. Action that is seriously intended to cause death
   d. Physical and social environment provided for the child
   e. Common household products that can be abused to achieve an altered state of consciousness
   f. Bodily dysfunctions that seem to have emotional and organic bases

2. Identify three interventions that may be used in the treatment of emotional or behavioral conditions. *(731)*

   a. _____

   b. _____

   c. _____

3. Creating an _____ environment is basic to all forms of therapy. *(731)*

4. List three signs of autism usually seen by 1 year of age. *(732)*

   a. _____

   b. _____

   c. _____

5.   What is the goal of therapy for a child who is autistic? *(732)*

_____

_____

_____

6.   What strategies can the nurse use when caring for a child with autism during hospitalization? *(732)*

_____

_____

7.   Describe the nurse's role in caring for a child with obsessive-compulsive disorder. *(732)*

_____

_____

8.   List five common signs and symptoms experienced by adolescents who are depressed. *(733)*

a.   _____

b.   _____

c.   _____

d.   _____

e.   _____

9.   The presence of which three factors increases the likelihood that a suicide attempt by an adolescent will be successful? *(733)*

a.   _____

b.   _____

c.   _____

10. Manifestations of suicidal behavior include: *(733)*

a.   _____

b.   _____

c.   _____

d.   _____

e.   _____

f.   _____

Answer as either true (T) or false (F).

11. The nurse must take every threat of suicide seriously. *(733)* _____

12. A nursing role related to suicide is the identification of at-risk adolescents. *(733)* _____

Student Name_____

13. State the four levels of substance abuse. *(733)*

    a. _____

    b. _____

    c. _____

    d. _____

14. What are the two types of drug dependence? *(733)*

    a. _____

    b. _____

15. List two strategies for the prevention of substance abuse. *(737)*

    a. _____

    _____

    b. _____

    _____

16. What is a gateway substance? *(735)*

    _____

17. The most significant consequence of heroin abuse is the increased risk of _____
    _____. *(737)*

18. Give two examples of each of the following clinical manifestations of a child with attention deficit hyper-
    activity disorder (ADHD). *(739)*

    a. Inattention: _____

    _____

    b. Impulsiveness: _____

    _____

    c. Hyperactivity: _____

    _____

19. Describe the management of ADHD. *(739)*

    _____

    _____

20. The nurse can help a family cope with ADHD by emphasizing the child's _____ rather than
    the _____. *(739)*

21. The primary symptom of anorexia nervosa is _____. *(740)*

22. List five of the possible body changes associated with anorexia nervosa. *(740)*

    a. _____

    b. _____

    c. _____

    d. _____

    e. _____

23. List some of the common behaviors of families of children with anorexia nervosa. *(740)*

_____

_____

24. Describe the eating habits of an adolescent with bulimia. *(740)*

_____

_____

25. Siblings of children with a long-term illness are at risk for developing _____
and _____. *(741)*

THINKING CRITICALLY

1. In what way should care be altered when caring for a child with asthma who is also diagnosed as having ADHD?

CASE STUDY

1. Nine-year-old Kyle has arrived at the same-day surgery unit for dental extractions. Kyle was diagnosed with autism when he was 3 years old.
   a. What factors might influence Kyle's reaction to this hospital experience?
   b. You will be admitting Kyle to the unit. What information specific to autism would you elicit from Kyle's mother during the admission process?
   c. His mother tells you that Kyle is very anxious about his surgery. What strategies will you use to interact with Kyle?
   d. After Kyle has been taken to the operating room, his mother says, "I don't understand why my other children seem to resent Kyle." What do you think is the reason for this? How would you respond to this statement?

APPLYING KNOWLEDGE

1. Discuss in class how an adolescent suspected of being suicidal should be interviewed.

2. List two nursing diagnoses associated with depression. Discuss in a group how nursing care should be implemented for these diagnoses.

3. Care for a child who is admitted to the hospital with an emotional disorder.

4. Interview the family members of a child with ADHD. What impact has this condition had on them, individually and as a family?

Student Name _____

REVIEW QUESTIONS

1. The risk of death increases in a suicidal adolescent when: *(733)*
   1. he is an only child.
   2. he has a learning disorder.
   3. he has a definite plan of action.
   4. his parents are divorced.

2. The nurse talking with school-age children about alcohol would explain this substance is known to be a: *(736)*
   1. sedative.
   2. opiate.
   3. stimulant.
   4. antidepressant.

3. Marijuana has which of the following physical effects? *(736)*
   1. Respiratory depression
   2. Pupil dilation
   3. Anorexia
   4. Tachycardia

4. The street name for a form of cocaine is: *(737)*
   1. crap.
   2. smack.
   3. hash.
   4. crack.

5. Primary to prevention of substance abuse in children is a: *(737)*
   1. positive self-image.
   2. strong religious belief.
   3. strict family.
   4. good education.

6. Adolescents who seek help for a substance abuse problem usually do so because: *(737)*
   1. there are no other options.
   2. they have friends in treatment.
   3. they realize they need help.
   4. their family encourages them.

7. If a nurse suspects an adolescent is contemplating suicide, he or she should: *(733)*
   1. avoid discussing the topic.
   2. ask the parents if they agree.
   3. ask the adolescent directly if he or she is thinking of killing him- or herself.
   4. observe him or her closely.

8. The best nursing response to a depressed adolescent is: *(733)*
   1. "Cheer up, things will get better."
   2. "Let's talk about how you are feeling."
   3. "Things always seem worse than they are."
   4. "You are lucky to have so many friends."

9. The type of drug dependence that causes withdrawal symptoms is called: *(733)*
    1. psychologic.
    2. pharmacologic.
    3. physical.
    4. mental.

10. Adolescents who drink even small amounts of alcohol are at increased risk to: *(734)*
    1. develop acne.
    2. become obese.
    3. have a drop in their intelligence.
    4. have an accident.

11. Bulimia is described as: *(740)*
    1. binge eating followed by self-induced vomiting.
    2. inability to eat due to fear of gaining weight.
    3. a systemic infection caused by a parasite.
    4. a secondary infection caused by a parasite.

12. A 16-year-old male who has broken off with his girlfriend threatens to kill himself. The nurse knows that this behavior: *(733)*
    1. is attention-seeking.
    2. should be taken seriously.
    3. should be ignored.
    4. is a normal reaction to the situation.

13. What is the most appropriate nursing response to a parent who states, "I hope my son outgrows his attention-deficit/hyperactivity disorder"? *(739)*
    1. "There are medications that can cure ADHD."
    2. "The symptoms decrease as the child matures."
    3. "Does anyone else in your family have ADHD?"
    4. "This is something that can continue into adulthood."

14. Children with ADHD: *(739)*
    1. may experience low self-esteem.
    2. are usually high achievers.
    3. usually have many friends.
    4. excel when given tasks that require intricate work.

15. An adolescent tells the nurse he has needed to increase his alcohol intake to feel its effect. The nurse recognizes that which situation has developed? *(733)*
    1. Psychological dependence
    2. Physical dependence
    3. Tolerance to the substance
    4. Withdrawal symptoms

CHAPTER 33
Complementary and Alternative Therapies in Maternity and Pediatric Nursing

Answer Key: Textbook page references are provided as a guide for answering these questions. A complete answer key was provided for your instructor.

LEARNING ACTIVITIES

1. Give examples of the following therapies. Can you identify examples other than those listed in the text? *(743)*

   a. Complementary therapy _____

   _____

   b. Alternative therapy _____

   _____

2. What is the current status of regulation and licensure in the United States related to complementary and/or alternative therapies? *(744)*

   _____

   _____

3. a. What conditions can massage therapy benefit? *(745)*

   _____

   b. What are contraindications for use of massage therapy? Why? *(745)*

   _____

   _____

4. a. What is the use of an acupressure wristband during pregnancy? *(746-747)*

   _____

   b. What acupoints should be avoided during pregnancy and why? *(746-747)*

   _____

   _____

5. What are cautions and potential risks of homeopathic medicines? *(747)*

   _____

   _____

6. a. List some essential oils that should not be used during pregnancy. *(748)*

   _____

   _____

   b. List oils that may be beneficial during pregnancy. What are their effects? *(748)*

   _____

   _____

   c. List essential oils that may benefit children with chronic pain. *(748)*

   _____

   _____

7. a. How is guided imagery believed to be therapeutic? *(748)*

   _____

   b. How can a nurse use guided imagery to help a woman in labor? *(748)*

   _____

   _____

8. List two problems in terms of regulation or control that the consumer encounters when using an herbal product. *(749)*

   a. _____

   b. _____

9. What are the cautions if herbal remedies are used during pregnancy, breastfeeding, or in children? *(749-751)*

   a. Use during pregnancy _____

   _____

   b. Use when breastfeeding _____

   _____

   c. Use in children _____

   _____

Student Name _____

10. List 11 herbs that a pregnant woman should not take. *(749)*

a. _____

b. _____

c. _____

d. _____

e. _____

f. _____

g. _____

h. _____

i. _____

j. _____

k. _____

11. Why should a pregnant woman avoid the herbs listed in question 10? *(749)*

_____

12. List four methods used as an alternative to hormone replacement therapy to manage the discomforts of menopause. *(750-751)*

a. _____

b. _____

c. _____

d. _____

APPLYING KNOWLEDGE

1. Choose a complementary or alternative therapy that you have heard of, used, or considered using. Go to the web site for the National Center for Complementary and Alternative Medicine at the National Institutes of Health at http://nccam.nih.gov/. Identify information about the uses, effectiveness, and adverse effects of the therapy you have chosen.

2. Attend a childbirth class in which preparation for labor is covered. What complementary therapies do you see taught to expectant parents in the class?

REVIEW QUESTIONS

1. What is the most important reason a nurse should ask specifically about use of complementary or alternative therapy when admitting a patient to the hospital? *(743-744)*
   1. Use of these therapies gives insight into the person's cultural background.
   2. Most therapies are promoted by those with little education in their use.
   3. Knowledge of possible interactions with prescribed traditional drugs reduces the chance of complications.
   4. The patient and family should be educated about the harmful effects of most complementary therapies.

2. A woman is troubled by hot flashes as she approaches menopause. She wants to avoid hormone replacement therapy because her mother had breast cancer and asks the nurse if natural remedies will help her. The best nursing response is that: *(750-751)*
   1. these discomforts are normal for menopause and will gradually go away as she ages.
   2. some herbs may help her symptoms but she should consult her physician before using them.
   3. most herbs are regulated by the Food and Drug Administration as estrogen would be regulated.
   4. heat therapy is the most reliable way to reduce nighttime hot flashes.

3. A 3-year-old child is hospitalized for pneumonia. The nurse notes marks on the abdomen and asks the parents about how the child received them. The parents reply that they often use "coin rubbing" when the child is ill. Based on this explanation, the nurse should: *(745-746)*
   1. document the marks and the parents' explanation for them.
   2. consult with child protective services because of possible abuse.
   3. explain to the parents that this practice cannot heal an infection.
   4. tell the parents that coin rubbing is dangerous to small children.

4. Energy therapy that may relieve nausea and vomiting associated with chemotherapy is: *(746)*
   1. effleurage of the abdomen.
   2. cold applied to the head.
   3. aromatherapy with essential oils and essences.
   4. transcutaneous electrical nerve stimulation.

5. A woman comes to clinic for her regular prenatal visit. She tells the nurse that acupressure has helped her with many discomforts, including the nausea she felt during early pregnancy. The best nursing response is: *(746-747)*
   1. acupressure on the bottom of her foot can help relieve the backache that often occurs during late pregnancy.
   2. acupuncture is safer than acupressure for relief of discomforts that are common during early and late pregnancy.
   3. several areas for pressure should be avoided during pregnancy to reduce the risk for preterm birth.
   4. it is best to avoid all types of unproven complementary therapies when she is pregnant.

6. When determining the dose of herbal therapy, the practitioner uses the: *(749)*
   1. person's body weight.
   2. person's age and sex.
   3. largest dose the person can tolerate.
   4. immune status of the person.

Student Name _____

7. A woman has taken a number of vitamins and herbal therapies throughout her pregnancy. To avoid infection while she is breastfeeding she takes large quantities of vitamin C. The nurse should advise the woman that: *(749)*
   1. vitamin C can reduce the chance of infection in both her and the baby.
   2. vitamin C is a fat-soluble vitamin and should not be taken in large doses.
   3. taking vitamin C with a milk product will enhance its absorption.
   4. colic is more likely in the baby if she takes large amounts of vitamin C.

8. A woman who is 30 weeks pregnant enjoys a sauna many times to help her relax after work. The nurse should advise her to: *(751)*
   1. keep the heat level low enough to avoid sweating.
   2. all heat therapy is contraindicated during pregnancy.
   3. she should leave the sauna if her pulse reaches 120.
   4. have another person with her when she uses the sauna.

CROSSWORD PUZZLE

Student Name _____

Across

4. Use of plants, herbs, and earth minerals to stimulate the body's immune system or help specific health problems *(747)*
5. Abbreviation for the agency that regulates drugs for effectiveness and safety *(745)*
9. Pathway to a specific organ or body part; used in acupuncture and acupressure *(746)*
10. Type of massage used during labor, often performed by the laboring woman *(745)*
14. Use of an electronic instrument to help a person recognize muscle tension *(749)*
18. Practitioner who combines traditional and manipulative therapy *(745-746)*
19. Stimulation of nerve cells using very thin needles *(746-747)*
22. Another name for traditional medicine *(745)*
23. Unconventional therapy that replaces mainstream therapy *(743)*
24. Mexican cultural folk healer *(744, Box 33-7)*

Down

1. Therapy delivered by suggestions given to a person when he/she is in a state of induced sleep *(748)*
2. Digitalis originates in this plant *(749)*
3. Nerve energy is thought to restore or maintain health; care involves the relationship between the spinal column and nervous system *(749)*
6. Hindu healing that considers the biological rhythms of nature *(747)*
7. Pressure, stretching, and manipulation of the fascia to increase muscle and bone function *(745)*
8. Acronym for electric current sent through the skin to stimulate nerves *(746)*
11. Use of water to promote relaxation *(748)*
12. Use of many medications *(745)*
13. Type of massage to relieve muscle tension and trigger points of pain *(745)*
15. Nontraditional therapy used in conjunction with conventional therapy *(743)*
16. Use of concentrated essential oils combined with steam or baths to inhale or bathe the skin *(748)*
17. Form of herbal remedy that contains a large quantity of alcohol *(749)*
20. Opiate drugs are related to this plant *(749)*
21. Finger pressure used to prevent disease *(747)*